Myofascial Relea

Myofascial Release Self-Treatment Guide.

Drug Free Methods and Tools to Stop Your Pain.

By

Robert Ryder

Table of Contents

4

About The Author

Robert Ryder is a retired doctor in Chicago, USA, specialized in physiotherapy and myofascial release. He has helped countless people, including athletes, with myofascial pain.

He has also suffered from myofascial pain himself, before specializing in treating it.

Some of his patients lived too far and couldn't travel to his practice often enough but still wanted to do myofascial release at home. That's how the idea of this book was born: to help people to treat trigger points at home. He has used his own medical knowledge and practice, as well as advice and success stories from his patients.

Introduction

If you have ever experienced unexplained pains that have no association with any specific disease, or you are unable to find the source of pain, believe me, you are not alone. Millions of people around the world are experiencing this scenario without any luck in treatments. These ailments are often neglected because of the confusion associated with them. Nearly every individual experiences unexplained pain at least once in his/her life. The financial burden associated with the treatment of these pains in some countries can be overwhelming, and unfortunately, the right diagnosis is often missed, leading to years of misery and frustration.

Correct diagnosis is the only key to successful treatment, treatment that doesn't involve surgery or an unending list of medicines and side effects associated with them. Most of the time, a positive change in posture or a simple massage at the right spot can alleviate the symptoms even in minutes. Finding the right spot and right source is essential, and failure in achieving this simple step leads to years of unresolved pains.

Myofascial pain is a collection of two words. "Myo" means muscle, and "Fascia" is a connecting structure between our muscles, skeleton, viscera, and skin. Fascia helps in coordinating our movements, and it helps in moving our body as a whole. Muscles help in initiating and controlling the movement while fascia provides the direction and harmony in our movements. It also supports our hollow structures, such as organs. So, the myofascial system of our body acts as a unit, and any issue associated with muscles can affect the fascia and vice versa.

Myofascial pain is not just a disease; it's a syndrome of a collection of different painful illnesses present in our muscles and fascial structures. The main reasons for myofascial pain syndromes are:
- poor posture
- inactivity
- muscle fatigue
- stress
- over-work
- mood disorders

- sleep disorders
- many autoimmune diseases in which the body's own immunity negatively affects the different organ systems.

Some examples of these diseases are rheumatoid arthritis and fibromyalgia. More than one issue can also be present together, which can increase the intensity and duration of pain in these individuals.

The right treatment of these myofascial pains involves a clear understanding of the involved structure, pathology of the issue, the right tools and skill-set, and a strong will to prevent the risk factors for recurrence. I have lived for years in this misery, as for most of the time my pains went unnoticed, and even I couldn't find the source of pain by myself. That led to a wrong diagnosis and I had to take a lot of medication, which had their own side effects. Until, I found about myofascial pain syndrome and terminologies like trigger points, tender points, fascial distortion, and myofascial slings.

To my surprise, nearly every myofascial pain could be cured through self-treatment. Sometimes a good massage at the tight band in the neck muscles helped me to treat the symptoms of my severe headaches.

I found out about the association between trigger points and traveling pain, which is by far the most common cause of myofascial pain. Some convenient tools also helped me to manage these pains on my own. In this book, I have tried to help you in mastering the art of self-treatment for nearly every cause of myofascial pain.

Myofascial pain is present in muscle or fascia and it can be due to trigger points, tender points, fascial distortion, etc. I have also provided important details about the involved structures in an easy way that will help you in understanding the pathological processes associated with myofascial pain.

Separate chapters are devoted to discussing different reasons for myofascial pain and self-treatment methods. The first part of the book includes the basic anatomy of muscle and fascia, history of myofascial release techniques, signs and symptoms of myofascial pain, pre-treatment and post-treatment guidelines, indications and contraindications of self-treatment, precautions, and limitations associated with self-treatments for myofascial pain.

The next segment of the book will tell you about a variety of different causes that are involved in myofascial pain.

The last part of the book involves a detailed discussion about self-treatments and preventions of myofascial pain.

Before you come to the main part in this book explaining treatment at home, it is essential that I explain the theory. If you understand how it all works, you have a much better chance to successfully do home treatments.

Glossary

Here is a quick summary and easy explanation of the terminology used in this book. All terms will be explained more in detail later.

Active stretching: You hold a position without any outside help, i.e. with your leg up in the air for around 10–15 seconds.

Arthritis: Arthritis is a term that refers to the pain and swelling in a joint.

Contractibility: Contractibility is the capacity of a muscle to shorten from a lengthened position.

Endurance: Endurance is the capability to maintain muscle's action for a prolonged period.

Fascia: Fascia is a very thin layer that wraps around your body, around every blood vessel, muscle, bone, organ and nerve. It covers the whole body from top to toe. It basically holds us together.

Fibromyalgia: In fibromyalgia, muscles of different body parts develop very painful, thick knots in them.

Flexibility: Flexibility is the ease of elongation in muscle after a contracted position.

IF: This device is very similar to TENS, but it is based on medium frequency currents. The use of the interferential device is proven in the case of myofascial pain and other neuromuscular injuries.

Isometric stretching: An isometric contraction is one without movement; this will give you a clue as to what this type of stretching consists of. You go to the end of the range of motion, contract your muscles, relax and repeat.

Lower cross syndrome: The muscles in the lower back and upper thighs/inguinal area get tight, while muscles in the abdomen and glutes get weak.

LTRPs: Latent trigger points are those that are perceived as a painful knot only after palpation.

Macronutrients: Macronutrients are the essential nutrients that comprise a more significant portion of our daily diet.

Micronutrients: This category of nutrients in our daily diet comprises of those salts, minerals, and vitamins which are present in food inherently or we can take them as a supplement.

Military posture: Military posture involves the straightening of the spine in the neck and lower back, which leads to severe tightness in these muscles.

Mindful breathing: In mindful breathing, you will be aware of inhalation, exhalation, depth of breathing, and frequency of breathing.

Muscle: Muscle is the contractile unit of the body that can contract and elongate.

Myofascial pain: Myofascial pain is a collection of two words "Myo" stands for muscle, and "fascia" is a connecting structure between our muscles, skeleton, viscera, and skin.

Posture: Posture is the alignment of our body in space. We possess different types of posture during our sitting, standing, or lying activities.

Power: Power is the capacity to contract in a given period forcefully. All the essential capabilities of a skeletal muscle are subject to change.

RA: Rheumatoid Arthritis affects non-weight bearing joints, and it is not a specific disease of the elderly population.

Rolfing: Rolfing is a massage technique proposed by Dr. Ida Rolf.

Sarcomere: The basic unit of a muscle is sarcomere.

Smooth muscles: Smooth muscles are present in the viscera, and they are not capable of voluntary contraction (i.e. we cannot control their contractions).

Static stretching: Static stretching focuses on increasing the range of motion by pushing beyond it whilst keeping the muscles fairly relaxed.

Swayback posture: In the swayback posture, our lumbar spine is slumped, leading to severe tightness in our lower back and front thigh muscle. Our abdominal and gluteal muscles are prone to weakness in this specific posture.

Tender points: These knots are different than the trigger points and are called tender points. On pressing these knots, pain in the involved muscle can be experienced, but this pain is not the referral pain (as in trigger points).

TENS: Transcutaneous Electrical Nervous Stimulation (TENS) is based on low-frequency currents, which help in managing pain related to nerves, muscles, and fascia.

Thera Cane: Thera Cane is a long tubular rod that has various extensions on it. One end of Thera Cane is U-shaped, which is also called the treatment zone because it is mostly used to treat the areas which are harder to reach otherwise.

TRPs: Trigger points are tight bands in muscles that have a characteristic knot in the middle.

Upper cross syndrome: The muscles of the upper back and front of the neck get weak, and the muscles of the chest and back of the neck get tight in upper cross syndrome.

Part 1) History, Anatomy, Sign, Symptoms and Causes.

1. Anatomy of Muscle

Muscle is the contractile unit of the body that can contract and elongate. The primary function of a muscle is to initiate and control movement. Our body is made up of smooth and skeletal muscles. Smooth muscles are present in the viscera, and they are not capable of voluntary contraction (i.e. we cannot control their contractions). Contractions and elongation of skeletal muscles can be controlled voluntarily, and myofascial pains are frequently associated with these muscles. Another classification of muscles is cardiac muscles, which are present in the heart. Cardiac muscles are also involuntary.

The basic unit of a muscle is sarcomere, and a muscle comprises of many small fibers. The fibers in muscles are wrapped in different sheets, which act as an anchor. A muscle contracts and relaxes in a uniform fashion, in which all fibers of a muscle are involved in a single movement. Protein is the essential building block of a muscle, and many nerves and blood vessels are also present in muscles.

The skeletal muscle has three parts; origin, insertion, and body. The origin of a muscle is the initial portion of a muscle from where it starts, and the area of attachment of that muscle with a bone is called insertion. The body of a muscle is the central, fleshy part between origin and insertion.

This basic anatomy of a muscle is critical because in muscle imbalances, some muscles get weaker while others become overly tight. Moreover, the trigger point (tight knots in a muscle) and tender points (painful round spots in the muscle associated with fibromyalgia) are present in the body of a muscle. These sites of muscles should be released to cure myofascial pain. This procedure of normalizing the structural integrity of a painful muscle and its associated fascia is called myofascial release. A muscle is attached with its corresponding fascia, which helps in integrating the movement pattern of different muscles and acts as an anchor.

2. Anatomy of Fascia

A fascia is an anchoring sheet around the muscle beneath the skin and the viscera of the body. Viscera are the hollow organs in our body, which perform specific functions (stomach, liver, etc.)
The primary function of a fascia is to provide an anchor in different structures of the body. Fascia is elastic, and it is named according to the associated structures.

Muscular fascia is present around muscles, while visceral fascia is present around the viscera. Superficial fascia anchors different layers of skin, while deep fascia anchors deeper structures of the body.

It is only recently that the medical world realizes the importance of fascia and how it can create chronic pain. Many doctors, even osteopaths and physiotherapists who obtained their degree over 20 years ago haven't really studied fascia in detail and therefore many don't know a lot about its importance or treatment. This is also the reason why lots of chronic pain is misdiagnosed and pain killers are prescribed whilst often the pain is caused by fascia problems and muscle knots.

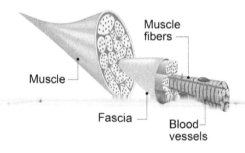

Fascia is a very thin layer that wraps around your body, around every blood vessel, muscle, bone, organ and nerve. It covers the whole body from top to toe and it basically holds us together.

The fascia determines our body posture and is designed to stretch when you move. Fascia should be slippery, smooth and easy to stretch, but it can become sticky and thick and this is what can create painful muscle knots, local pains and tightness that you can release at home. The aim of myofascial release is to restore the sticky fascia back to smooth.

Fascia is made up of collagen and fibroblasts, which help in maintaining the integrity of fascial sheaths. Muscle is more flexible than fascia, but twisting is more often encountered in fascial structures. The fascia is a very dense gel that can be molded and stretched only with slow and sustained pressure. The fibroblasts inside the gel respond positively to slow stretching by secreting chemicals that accelerate the healing process in the tissue around them.

Look at fascia as cling film. You can see on the picture below that it is smooth and easy to stretch.

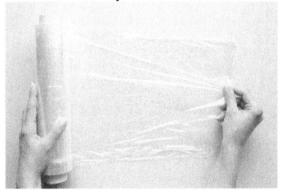

Bad posture, inactivity and inflammation are only a few reasons why your fascia can look as shown on the picture below: no longer smooth. If you have ever tried it, you know how difficult it is to make a piece of cling film back to being smooth, once it has been squashed together. Myofascial release does just that: turning sticky fascia that created muscle knots back into smooth fascia, releasing the pain the sticky fascia caused.

Cling film that has been pinched or squashed in different places will no longer do the job it's supposed to do: cover a plate of food. Instead, the edges of the plate won't be covered as the film has shrunk.

In a fibromyalgia patient, the fascia often feels and even looks (you can see the bumps in the muscles) like the cling film on the picture

below: not smooth at all, full of "pinched" cling film or in a fibromyalgia body: full of muscle knots.
If not treated, the muscle knots can get worse and sometimes so bad that another muscle tries to compensate and doing a job it is not designed to do. So as the cling film no longer does the job; the muscle no longer does the job either and is mal-functioning.

More and more muscle knots can appear, all over the body. This is one of the reasons why fibromyalgia patients often describe their pain as: "pain all over my body". Important to note that most of the time muscle knots are not the only problem in people with fibromyalgia as it is complex condition.

Any blunt or twisting force can tangle the fascia of the body, and this distortion can lead to unexplained pain in associated areas. A patient recognizes the fascial pain as dull, throbbing, and hard to localize, and it can be felt like trapped all under the skin. If a patient has many muscle knots, the pain can become severe. Any cause of pain in the muscle can lead to fascial pain and vice versa. Myofascial pain is discomfort associated with a muscle, fascia or both. A detailed history of the direction and nature of a blunt force or twisting movement can provide important information about the distortion in fascial sheets of the involved area.

Several manual therapies provide just the right amount and type of pressure needed to stimulate the fibroblasts and loosen those tight and dense areas. The primary one I recommend is myofascial release (MFR), a combination of sustained manual traction and prolonged gentle stretching. Studies show that the gentle, sustained pressure of myofascial release speeds up tissue healing and reduces inflammation.

Standard massage techniques do *not* stimulate fibroblasts or address fascial tightness, which may be why many people with fibromyalgia don't find much benefit from standard massage therapy.

Fascia Lines
There are main fascia lines within our body, and all of these are connected.

The main fascia lines are:
- Superfascial Front Line
- Superfascial Back Line
- Laterline Line
- Spiral Line
- Functional Line
- Arm Lines
- Diagonal Fascia Line

For a very detailed look at these, I recommend you read the book "*Myofascial Trains*" by Thomas W. Myers.
As all fascia lines are connected to each other, it could be that you are releasing a muscle knot in your upper lateral thigh and you actually feel a referred pain in your lateral calf. If you have a muscle knot in one fascia line, it will affect the proper functioning of the whole line.

In the diagonal fascia line, it could be that you have a muscle knot or ache in your upper right arm and you have referred pain in your left calf. You can conclude that fascia and muscle knots are not always easy to treat when you have several muscle knots in your body.

Releasing one knot can actually create new muscle knots to appear anywhere else in your body, because of these fascia lines. The whole fascia line needs to be knot free and smooth to function optimally. However, there are many people with muscle knots that don't actually have any pain but in most cases, the posture of these people will somehow be affected as the stuck fascia pulls on muscles and surrounding ligaments.

The fascia lines are also the reason why it can take several weeks or months before you can release all the muscle knots, if you have many. This is especially so for fibromyalgia patients who usually have a lot of muscle knots, all over their body.

Before you start your myofascial release, it is important that you self-educate on these fascia lines, as writing in detail about these would fill another book. Knowledge is power: power to carry out your treatment better and become totally pain free.

3. History of Myofascial Release Techniques

Myofascial pain has forever affected the lives of human beings. The treatment for myofascial pain was never hard to find, as the instinct behaviors of humans against the painful stimuli helped man to alleviate the pain. I can confidently say that the oldest myofascial release technique for myofascial pain is "massage". It involves the rubbing of a painful site either by the hands or with the help of a tool. Massaging the painful area is a part of instinct behavior against the pain.

Heat is another ancient technique to alleviate myofascial pain, because it helps in relaxing the painful and tight soft tissues in the involved area. Many ancient documents proved the use of heat as first-class treatment of myofascial pain syndrome. The use of different objects to press and release the tight soft tissues was also a common practice in very ancient human civilizations.

As time evolved, the understanding of myofascial pain syndromes became more transparent, and many new treatments were discovered to prevent and treat myofascial pain. The causes of myofascial pain were a common interest among different schools of thought in medicine. Osteopaths, chiropractors, and physiotherapists made most of the contributions to understanding the mechanism of myofascial pain and to propose the most effective treatments in these scenarios. Manual therapy is the latest field that has evolved in the art of myofascial release to a very advanced level.

The most common techniques of manual therapy for myofascial release are trigger band release, ischemic compression technique, cross-friction, and transverse massage; dry needling; gross, specific, and active isolated stretching; RICE technique; and the use of electrical and manual tools for myofascial releases. Fortunately, most of these techniques can be used as self-treatment of myofascial pain. I will describe some of these self-management techniques later.

4. Signs and Symptoms of Myofascial pain

The biggest issue associated with myofascial pain is the poorly localized pain pattern. When I was unaware of myofascial sources of unexplained pains, I tried a variety of medicines for differential diagnosis of my pains, which provided little to no benefits against my condition. After getting enough knowledge about myofascial pain and myofascial release, I realized that the pain was always associated with a source. Still, that source was not always present at the site of pain. Trigger points have a characteristic traveling pain, and every muscular trigger point has its referral zone.

I often suffered from headaches, and I could feel that there was something wrong in my neck. I realized that the knots in my neck muscles (trigger points) caused the referred pain in my head. Treating these tight knots in my neck muscles alleviated the pain in my head, and it was shocking for me. I concluded that the right knowledge about the signs and symptoms of myofascial pains was essential to making a correct diagnosis, and it helped me to plan the right treatment against the cause of my pains.

The most common signs and symptoms which can help in identifying the myofascial source of pain are:
1. Presence of a painful tight knot in a muscle (trigger point or tender point).
2. Traveling pain (also called referring pain) after pressing this knot (trigger point).
3. Dull and throbbing pain.
4. Hard to localize the actual source of pain (distorted fascia).
5. Feeling like some air is entrapped beneath the involved area (fascial distortion).
6. Pain during specific movements.
7. Joint pain (fibromyalgia and arthritis).
8. Restless Legs.
9. Unexplained headache.
10. Early fatigue.
11. Severe and frequent muscle cramps.

12. Feeling like the involved area is burning.
13. Numbness in the involved area.
14. Pain while stretching a specific muscle.
15. Inability to move a muscle to its complete range.
16. Swelling in the involved muscle.
17. Pain increases with activity.
18. Pain that relieves after rest (pain from systemic sources is mostly unchanged after rest).
19. Sweating in the involved area
20. Tight band in the involved muscle

These hallmarks are often present in the form of clusters, and it is also possible that more than one pathology is causing your myofascial pain. A patient having fibromyalgia often complains about joint pain as well as round, painful nodules in specific muscles of the body. A migraine patient can have very painful tight knots in their neck muscles. A blunt or twisting force on the arm can cause fascial distortion in that area, which is characterized by numbness, poorly localized and throbbing pain. So, careful consideration of the presenting symptoms can help in finding the actual cause of myofascial pain, and self-treatments can address those symptoms very effectively.

5. Pre and Post-Treatment Guidelines
A well-planned and mastered self-treatment protocol to manage myofascial pain can save time, money, and effort. Self-administered myofascial release techniques can treat nearly every type of myofascial pain. However, some important guidelines should always be kept in mind before and after administering the treatment for myofascial pain. Here, I will discuss only general self-treatment guidelines, which should be followed during every type of self-administered myofascial release technique. However, the specific pre, intra, and post-treatment guidelines of a targeted self-administered myofascial release technique are discussed in this book.

Pre-treatment guidelines
1. Although warming up your muscles is not a necessity, myofascial release often works better after warming up. Fascia loves being warm and is treated easier when warm.

You can warm up by either doing some light exercises or stretches, go for a walk or have a warm bath.
2. Always focus on the specific signs and symptoms of a targeted myofascial pain.
3. Find the actual cause of the targeted myofascial pain, which can reproduce the symptoms after triggering.
4. Find the most suitable and effective self-treatment for the targeted myofascial pain.
5. Find the associated indications/contraindications of selected self-treatment.
6. Revise all the necessary steps of self-treatment to administer it correctly.
7. Gather the necessary tools.
8. Place yourself in a comfortable position.
9. The targeted muscle/fascia should be as relaxed as possible.
10. Carefully control the intensity, duration, and frequency of the treatment.
11. Always cross-check the validity and suitability of your treatment to avoid any injury.
12. You should reach the targeted area comfortably.
13. Use the mirror when possible, because it increases the mind-body connection.
14. Always focus your mind on the treatment, because it increases the relaxation in targeted muscle/fascia.
15. Breathe normally while applying the self-treatment.
16. Where needed, you should ask someone to help you in administering the treatment.
17. If more than one issue is involved in triggering the targeted myofascial pain, address all the issues in the same sitting.
18. If addressing all the primary factors in the same session is overwhelming, try to stick to your comfort zone.
19. Ensure to take essential measures to avoid any discomfort.

Post-treatment guidelines
1. Always check the difference in signs and symptoms after administering the self-treatment.
2. The self-treatment should not increase the pain.
3. If treatment-induced pain persists for more than 24 hours, try to reduce the intensity of the treatment session.
4. If it doesn't help, always consult your doctor.

5. If the symptoms go unchanged even after 24 hours of administering the self-treatment, check for the applicability of your treatment technique.
6. Always allow your muscle/fascia to relax after the treatment session. Post-treatment stretching is usually beneficial.
7. Never over-treat your targeted area.
8. Fluid intake after the session can ease the pain.
9. Post-treatment breathing exercises help in normalizing the breathing pattern.
10. Expect some soreness in the area of the muscle knot you have released. This doesn't happen all the time but is perfectly normal, as the muscle and surrounding areas have to adjust.
11. Always stretch the muscle of the area you've treated e.g. if you have released a muscle knot in your upper arm, stretch the arm for a few seconds.

6. Indications and Contra-indications

Every treatment comes with its indications and contraindications. Careful consideration of these factors is essential to achieve post-treatment success. If you try to press a very painful muscle, it can increase the pain. Similarly, over-stretching a muscle can harm a tight muscle. I have discussed treatment-specific indications and contraindications in relevant sections. Still, in this section, I am describing the general factors, which can help you to decide your self-treatment plan for myofascial pain.

Indications
1. The treatment is easy to administer by the patient.
2. The treatment is easy to understand by the patient.
3. The tools involved in self-treatment are available.
4. The patient can quickly master the tools involved in self-treatment.
5. Self-treatment has proven benefits against the targeted tissue.
6. Self-treatment has very little to low side effects.
7. There are very little risks associated with the tools used for self-treatment.
8. The targeted area is easily approachable by the patient.
9. The patient doesn't possess other illnesses that can counteract with the targeted treatment.

10. Self-treatment doesn't involve dangerous positions which can lead to catastrophes.
11. Self-treatment doesn't require any particular license before practicing.

Contraindications
1. There are numerous chances that self-treatment can increase the pain in a patient.
2. The patient is not trained enough for the self-administration of targeted treatment.
3. The tools required for self-treatment are unavailable.
4. There are frequent side effects associated with targeted self-treatment or assistive tools.
5. The tools involved in self-treatment can be costly.
6. Your doctor has forbidden the self-treatment protocols because of valid reasons.
7. The treatment can interfere with the other illnesses of the patient.
8. Self-treatment is associated with more harm than benefits in your case.
9. Self-treatment has failed to treat the symptoms even if its applicability is well-established.

7. Precautions and Limitations
Self-treatment of myofascial pain usually provides beneficial results, but it is a smart idea to take all the necessary precautions. Moreover, there are several limitations in administering self-treatment for targeted myofascial pathology. In my case, I sometimes found it hard to approach the targeted muscle for self-treatment. Initially, I tried to approach it anyway, but it leads to postural injuries in my otherwise healthy muscles. So, it is my honest advice to check all the necessary precautions and limitations before applying self-treatment for myofascial pain disorders.

Precautions
1. Always ensure the safety protocols before the self-treatment of a targeted area.
2. Never use contaminated or worn-out tools for self-treatment.
3. If you don't know much about the efficacy of targeted self-treatment, it is better to do some research before applying it.

4. If you have serious pathologies like asthma, heart diseases, etc. then self-treatment of painful areas can increase the symptoms of these diseases.
5. If the signs and symptoms of a nodule are not consistent with a musculoskeletal origin, a detailed examination from your doctor should be your priority. A nodule is different than a myofascial trigger point or tender point. It is felt like a lump beneath the skin, and it can have non-musculoskeletal origins like cancer, infection, etc.
6. Patients with deep vein thrombosis should avoid massage or heating at the calf muscles because it can prove deadly.
7. If you have diabetes or you have an impaired sense of heat/cold, self-treatments that involve such modalities are prohibited for you.
8. If you have balance issues and self-treatment requires equilibrium, you should take necessary precautions to avoid falls.
9. The very old population and children should never be allowed to do self-treatment.
10. Pregnant females should take all the necessary precautions.

Limitations
1. Self-treatment requires a lot of training on your end.
2. Self-treatment can increase the pain when the technique is poor.
3. Not every area of the body is easily targeted for self-treatment.
4. Some tools are very costly or unavailable in some countries.
5. It is not a suitable option for older, pediatric, and mentally ill patients.
6. Bed-ridden patients have limitations for self-treatment.
7. Diagnosis is a bit tricky for self-treatment.
8. It is hard to decide which treatment is safer and more beneficial.
9. Some techniques of myofascial release require the support of a professional.

8. Tips for Family Members
Self-treatment of targeted myofascial pathology can easily be carried out with the proper technique. Some assistive tools help us to

administer the myofascial release technique to the targeted area properly.

I am going to describe some essential guidelines for family members, who can assist a patient in the self-administration of myofascial release technique for his/her myofascial pain syndromes. These guidelines will also help the family members to understand the process of disease and treatment better. Moreover, it will also help in the active engagement of family in the self-treatment of common myofascial pain problems.

Some specific guidelines for the families of patients are:
1. The family should encourage the patient to actively learn and administer the treatments for myofascial pain at home.
2. The family should be involved as an active stakeholder in the self-treatment of the patient's myofascial problems.
3. The availability of private space for the self-treatment of myofascial pathologies is the family's responsibility.
4. Help the patient in self-treatment when required.
5. Help with the availability of necessary tools when patients are unable to get them alone.
6. Always ask and support the patient about the progress made during self-treatment.
7. Encourage the patient to maintain the correct posture all day long to avoid the recurrence of myofascial problems.
8. Encourage the patient to consult a competent doctor if self-treatment provides little or no improvements.

9. Common Reasons for Myofascial pain

I have tried to explain all the necessary guidelines about the self-treatment of myofascial pain. This important part of the book is about the common reasons associated with myofascial pain. Myofascial pain affects all types of people. It neither spares athletes nor sedentary adults. The top 12 causes of myofascial pain are listed below.

Faulty posture
Posture is the alignment of our body in space. We possess different types of posture during our sitting, standing, or lying activities. The ideal posture is the one in which our muscles are most relaxed and

safe from tightness or weakness. Faulty postures cause severe strains on our soft tissues (muscles, ligaments, tendons, and fascia).

The association between trigger points and faulty posture is well-established, and the most prevalent population having myofascial pain comprises those individuals who possess faulty postures. In the forward neck posture, our neck and upper back are slouched, which leads to tightness in the muscles of the back of the neck and chest. The muscles of the middle back and front of the neck are prone to weakness in this specific posture.

In the swayback posture, our lumbar spine is slumped, leading to severe tightness in our low back and front thigh muscle. Our abdominal and gluteal muscles are prone to weakness in this specific posture.

Military posture involves the straightening of the spine in the neck and lower back, which leads to severe tightness in these muscles. Many people use mobile phones and laptops in the faulty neck postures, leading to myofascial pain in the neck muscles.

In this digital era, people spend most of their time sitting on couches and doing nothing but browsing their cell phones in a faulty posture, which is one of the leading causes of myofascial pains and discomforts.

Inactivity
Our body is not designed to sit for 8 hours a day. It is designed to move for ultimate functioning. Our skeletal muscles possess five characteristics; flexibility, contractibility, strength, endurance, and power.

- Flexibility is the ease of elongation in muscle after a contracted position.
- Contractibility is the capacity of a muscle to shorten from a lengthened position.
- Strength is the capability to generate force against an imposed load.
- Endurance is the capability to maintain muscle's action for a prolonged period.

- Power is the capacity to contract in a given period forcefully. All the essential capabilities of a skeletal muscle are subject to change.

These five abilities of skeletal muscles severely decline in inactive and sedentary people because a variety of exercises and training is essential to optimize these qualities of a muscle. The tightened muscles often develop tight, painful knots in them. Weak muscles are over-stretched, which also involves associated fascia, and myofascial pains in these muscles are also widespread. These inactive muscles are also subject to early fatigue, which is a leading cause of myofascial pain syndrome in the inactive population.

Muscle fatigue
Malnutrition and inactivity are the leading causes of fatigue in muscles. These muscles cannot keep up with the activities of daily life, which leads to an increased prevalence of muscle knots and myofascial slings in these muscles. Fatigability is also induced by poor posture and over-work.

Forceful contractions
I can remember an incident when I was about to drop my phone; I forcefully contracted my bicep muscle to hold it firmly. It was my innate response, but the result was devastating. I saved the phone but suffered severe pain in my bicep muscle for more than one week. During that time, I was unaware of myofascial pain or myofascial release, so I tried a variety of medications without any luck of improvement.

I had to see a therapist, who found a trigger point in my bicep muscle. When she pressed that tight knot, I experienced the same traveling pain. A forceful and uncontrolled contraction causes fascial distortion in that specific area, as well as possible muscle knots in involved muscles.

Over-stretching
Much like a forceful contraction, an uncontrolled stretch in muscle also inhibits the elongation of a muscle, and the result is fascial distortion and myofascial pain. Many cross-country athletes and

professional runners often experience myofascial pain because of over-stretched muscles.

Fibromyalgia

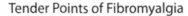

Tender Points of Fibromyalgia

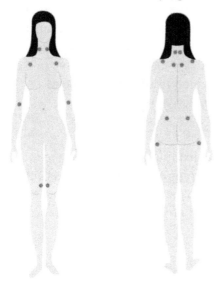

This disease affects millions of people around the world, and it is recognized by the presence of persistent pain in muscles and even in joints (rare). In fibromyalgia, muscles of different body parts develop very painful thick knots in them. These knots are different than the trigger points and are called tender points. On pressing these knots, pain in the involved muscle can be experienced, but this pain is not the referral pain (as in trigger points). I have described the specific characteristics and treatments of tender points in the relevant section.

Trigger points
I have already discussed trigger points earlier in this book and will discuss more later. As a reminder: visit www.triggerpoints.net to find where to do self-treatment.

Arthritis
Age-related or autoimmune diseases of joints that cause damage in joint surfaces are termed as arthritis. Osteoarthritis is age-related wear and tear in weight-bearing joints, while rheumatoid arthritis is an autoimmune disease that also involves young adults. Rheumatoid

arthritis patients always present one or more trigger points, and the prevalence of myofascial pain in these patients is very high. In osteoarthritis patients, abnormal loading in muscles of weight-bearing areas leads to severe myofascial pains and fascial distortions.

Faulty biomechanics
Biomechanics is the study of human motions. It is a term usually associated with athletes. Active individuals, especially the athletic populations, have to spend hours in training for a specific sport. However, if their form is poor or their muscles are not well-trained for that specific athletic activity, nothing can stop them from developing myofascial pain problems. These individuals are the perfect candidates for self-treatment for myofascial pain problems. Moreover, a detailed biomechanical assessment of their athletic form is also very essential to prevent these issues.

Over-activity
Inactivity is hazardous for the muscles and fascia of the body. Over-activity is the overuse of a muscle(s), and it is also harmful to the soft tissues of the body. Myofascial pain syndromes are very common among people who spend hours in front of a computer. Any type of over-activity (posture-related, exertion-related, or training-related) can lead to myofascial pain syndrome. Fatigability is the main factor behind the myofascial pains in these populations.

Stress and anxieties
Every-day stress is, by far, the most common cause of myofascial pain in otherwise healthy individuals. Stress can be due to work overload, or it can occur as a result of some painful event. Whatever the cause of stress, myofascial pains in these patients are unstoppable; people with long-term stress disorders present severe tightness in the neck and head muscles. Headaches, trigger points, and other myofascial issues are very common in these patients. Anxieties, especially social anxieties, are also the leading cause of myofascial pain syndrome.

People who have had trauma in their past can have muscle knots that have been there for many years. As the body learns to adjust and moves using surrounding muscles, it could be that you haven't even felt the knots. However, at some time in your life, your body might create pain around the knots. These type of muscle knots are usually more difficult to treat but not impossible.

Sleep disturbances
People suffering from sleep-related disorders such as insomnia, excessive sleep, and vivid dreams often present with severe tightness in the neck and head muscles. These people show early signs of fatigue and mood irritations. The cumulative effects of all these disorders lead to severe myofascial pain issues in this population.

10. Risk Factors for Myofascial Pain

A risk factor is a term associated with those characteristics in a person that can lead to a specific type of disease. Smoking is the biggest culprit behind lung cancer. Eating junk food is a risk factor for obesity. Excessive alcohol consumption is the most significant risk factor for liver failure. Similarly, many risk factors are also associated with myofascial pain. Addressing these risk factors first handed helps in the prevention of myofascial pain. It also helps in controlling the recurrence of symptoms after a successful self-treatment. I thought it imperative that I tell you about these risk factors in detail.

1. People with lots of stress, trauma or PSTD, together with overworked people, are more at risk.
2. There are a lot of people who have an inactive lifestyle and don't get muscle knots at all. It is a contributing factor.
3. Substance abuse and smoking negatively affects the muscles and other soft tissue so, these are also significant risk factors for myofascial pain.
4. Unhealthy relationships trigger stress and depression, so they can directly link with myofascial pain.
5. Some people have natural tendencies to develop painful knots in their muscles.
6. The presence of comorbid factors such as diabetes, heart diseases, liver disorders, arthralgia (joint issues), myalgia (muscle pathologies), migraines, spinal disc issues, pathologies related to nerves, and depressive disorders are often present with myofascial pain problems.
7. Old age and the female gender are also significant risk factors for myofascial pain.

8. Bed-ridden patients are at the risk of developing severe issues in muscle, fascia, and other soft/hard tissues of the body.
9. School children who have to carry heavy bags are often presented with myofascial issues.
10. Labor and office workers who have increased exposure to fatigue are among those populations who have the highest numbers of myofascial pain problems.
11. Pregnancy itself is a risk factor because the body undergoes drastic changes in these months. These changes are not in favor of myofascial structures of the body. Weight distribution among muscles and ligaments is severely compromised, especially in more than six months pregnant females. Moreover, the supportive skeleton of the body is badly disturbed in pregnant individuals. All these factors cause accumulative damages to muscles and fascia, leading to myofascial pain problems.
12. An inactive lifestyle is the most significant risk factor, which can lead to persistent myofascial pain.

PART 2) An In-depth Look at Causes

I have discussed all the basic factors associated with myofascial pain. The basic anatomy of muscle and fascia is very important to understand the pathological processes of myofascial pain. The risk factors associated with myofascial pain syndromes should be managed in the first place to prevent the occurrence of complications. It is necessary to be aware of the important causes of myofascial pain syndromes.

Lots of techniques can be utilized to manage myofascial pain syndromes, but there are several limitations in managing myofascial pain at home. However, these limitations can easily be covered by utilizing the right tools and skills.

In this portion of the book, I am going to discuss some very important causes of myofascial pain syndromes. The biggest challenge in myofascial pains is finding the source of pain. Sometimes these types of pains are dull and poorly localized, which makes it hard to understand the pattern of pain. The true source of myofascial pain can be hidden in a sore muscle, or it can be the distorted fascia.

Some people feel a sharp pain in muscles after lifting a heavy object, and this can also involve the associated tendons and fascia. Athletes (especially combat sports athletes) are very prone to myofascial pain syndromes because of faulty biomechanics. Muscle spasm is also a hidden cause of myofascial pain syndrome.

Another important but very underrated cause of myofascial pain syndrome is the entrapment of nerves in different areas. Old injuries (accidents, falls, etc.) can cause fascial distortion, which can cause myofascial pain of a poorly localized nature.

This portion of the book will provide a detailed insight into all these hidden causes of myofascial pain syndromes. By reading and memorizing these pathologies, you will be able to identify the main reason behind your myofascial pain correctly, and it will help you to understand those pathologies more precisely.

1. Postural Abnormalities

Posture refers to the body's position either in standing, sitting, or lying. It involves a true sense of position in space, and our muscles and skeleton help us to adopt different postures. There are different postures in standing, sitting, and lying; however, a person should adopt a correct posture to avoid any musculoskeletal pathology.

The question "what is an ideal posture?" has confused many health professionals for centuries, and now, it is well-established that there is no single ideal posture. It is a dynamic state of the human body that should be adjusted according to the needs and requirements. For example, if a soldier is standing in an erect posture for more than an hour; he/she has to be relaxed and adopt a more slouched posture for the rest of the day to avoid strain on his/her low back and neck muscles. Similarly, if a person is standing in a slouched posture with round shoulders and a forward neck, he/she has to adjust his posture to a more erect one after 15-20 minutes because this slouched posture can cause severe strain on his/her neck and back muscles. In another example, if a person is sitting upright for more than 20 minutes, he/she has to be more reclined on his chair afterwards to avoid strain on the body.

So, you can have an idea from the above examples that the posture is a dynamic state, and it has to be changed more frequently. A prolonged upright standing posture is as dangerous as a slouched and forward neck posture. Let's discuss some important postures and associated pathologies that can cause myofascial pain syndromes.

Standing posture

In an anatomical or more natural standing posture, a person should have straight shoulders, an upright neck, a straight back, and good control of their lower extremities. The arms should be at the side of the body, and every muscle should be as relaxed as possible. However, it is hard to maintain a perfect standing posture, and many people fail to perceive the correct standing posture because of muscle imbalances in their neck, upper, or even lower back. Moreover, a weak lower extremity can also disturb a standing posture. Some faulty standing postures are listed below.

Swayback posture

This is also called the lazy posture because the person stands with hips tucked in, slouched back and forward neck. It causes severe strain on muscles that are present on the back of the neck. It also causes tightness in the lower back muscles. The person possessing the swayback posture is very prone to myofascial pains because of severe strains and abnormalities in their muscles. These people also possess less control over their postural muscles when they get weaker with time, and this issue can lead to myofascial pain in the back and neck.

Military posture

In this posture, a person stands upright with a stiff back and neck. When this posture is adopted for a prolonged period of time, it causes severe strains on the neck, middle, and lower back muscles, leading to postural instabilities, muscle tightness, and eventually, myofascial pain syndromes. Another issue with the military posture is the entrapment of a nerve called the scapular nerve beneath the scapula (bone of the middle back), which is perceived as a dull pain in the middle back, more towards the right/left side of the spine.

Even massage and self-release of tight muscles of the middle back cannot provide relief to this type of myofascial pain because the cause is not present in the muscles. However, proper neurodynamics (exercises to improve mobility of nerves) can cure this issue. Now, you can understand how a proper diagnosis can lead to a more successful outcome in the case of myofascial pain syndrome.

Lower cross syndrome

This syndrome is a cluster of problems present around the pelvic region. This is mostly associated with the standing posture. In a prolonged faulty standing posture, some muscles get tight while others get weak. This muscle imbalance leads to poorly localized myofascial pains in the back, neck, legs, pelvis, and even in the abdomen. It is called a cross syndrome because of muscles appearing in the crossed form are involved.

The muscles in the lower back and upper thighs/inguinal area get tight, while muscles in the abdomen and glutes get weak. This muscle imbalance also leads to walking instabilities and, thus, more risks of myofascial pain syndrome. The tight muscles are more prone to develop myofascial pains because of prolonged strains on these muscles.

Sitting posture

The perfect sitting posture requires an upright back, arms at the side of the body, and an upright neck. Eyes should be facing forward. Legs should be relaxed, and the angle at the hips should be 90 degrees. It is important to relax your muscles maximally. However, it is hard to maintain a perfect sitting posture, and many people are habitual to adopting a more relaxed and slouched posture, which can lead to myofascial pain syndromes.

Slouched sitting posture

In a slouched sitting posture, the neck is forward, shoulders are round and tucked in towards the chest, the upper and middle back is also round, and there is more strain on the lower back. This posture causes severe strain on the posterior neck and upper back muscles. The prevalence of myofascial headaches in people who are habitual to slouched sitting is much higher.

Over-straight sitting posture

This is also called the anxious posture because it is mostly observed in confused and anxious people. Have you ever faced anxiety during an interview? If yes, then you can recall the tight feeling in the neck as you are glued to the chair and could barely move. In an overly straight sitting posture, the neck and back are very tight, and arms are pressed with the torso. The legs are also pressed together, and feet are pressed to the ground. Nearly every muscle of the body is tight in this posture, and if it is maintained for a prolonged period, the risk of myofascial pain syndromes increases to many folds. This posture is as dangerous as the slouched sitting posture, and it can also cause entrapment of the scapular nerve.

Upper cross syndrome

As we previously discussed, lower cross syndrome is present around the pelvis. Upper cross syndrome is present around the neck. It is also characterized by the crossed appearance of pathological muscles. The muscles of the upper back and front of the neck get weak, and the muscles of the chest and back of the neck get tight in upper cross syndrome. This syndrome is the characteristic sign of the forward head posture in which the neck is forward, the chin is tucked, and shoulders are round. The upper cross syndrome is the main reason for myofascial pains in the neck, upper back, and chest area. It is also the main cause of the headache and related myofascial pains in the areas of skull and eyes.

Lying posture

Believe me or not, the biggest culprit of most myofascial pain is an abnormal lying posture. Lying is often thought of as the most relaxed position of the body, but if the lying posture is not good, you will be putting abnormal strain on many muscles for more than 6 hours during your sleep cycle. The reason for most severe myofascial pains after waking up is because of prolonged strain on associated muscles in the lying posture. An ideal posture can be straight lying or lying on the side of your body, but the key is, every muscle of your body should be as relaxed as possible.

Many physicians and physiotherapists prescribe special pillows that aid in a relaxed neck posture during sleep. Pillows at the sides of your back help in keeping the strains away from your middle and lower back, while pillows between the thighs or below knees can help in minimizing strain on your lower extremities during sleep. The quality and type of mattress are also very important when it comes to a proper sleeping posture. A hard or springy mattress is a personal choice, and the best sleeping mattress is the one that imposes minimum stain to the back and neck.

During sleep, water is also redistributed in the body, and spinal discs also absorb much of this water. Muscles regenerate during sleep, and the growth hormone releases in the deepest phase of sleep. If the lying posture is not optimal, it affects the sleep cycle, which in turn leads to severe myofascial pains such as headaches, myofascial trigger points, joint pains, etc. Moreover, any abnormal or jerky movement during sleep (because of a vivid dream, etc.) can also lead to severe myofascial pain and fascial distortions.

So, the above discussion about posture can provide great insight into different types of perfect and faulty postures. Knowing your posture and constant awareness of your body positioning is very important if you want to prevent myofascial pain syndromes. I will discuss important self-treatments to correct postural misalignments and muscular strains related to faulty postures.

2. Sleep Disorders

Sleep is a state of the body in which our mind is as relaxed as possible, and there is a very low tone in every muscle of the body. Sleep is our built-in state of rest, and our body heals itself during the deepest phases of sleep. Sleep is divided into different phases, and the deepest phase of sleep is called rapid eye movement, in which dreams occur. It is essential to go into this deepest phase of sleep if we want to avoid myofascial pain syndromes. The reason is a growth hormone that is released in this deepest phase of sleep. The growth hormone causes growth in children, and in adults, it is important to heal the all-day-long strains and stresses imposed on our muscles and joints.

Unfortunately, 1 in 3 people around the globe suffer from sleep disorders. Every person suffers from sleep issues in his/her life, but the myofascial pains are most prevalent in those people who have prolonged disturbances in their sleep cycle. These sleep disorders can be due to anxieties, depression, addictions, work-overload, traumas, and environmental factors. Chronic illnesses or acute pains also significantly impair the quality of sleep.

The lying posture should be optimal, and every muscle should be as relaxed as possible for a night of quality sleep. Moreover, the sleep cycle should be around 6-8 hours, however this varies per person. People try to take naps rather than a full 6-8 hours of sleep, but this practice makes them prone to myofascial pain syndromes because the muscles cannot get enough rest to heal themselves.

Disturbed sleep causes pressure on the head and neck muscles, leading to myofascial pain syndromes in these areas. Moreover, it also causes strains in back muscles, leading to muscle imbalances and postural instabilities. Studies have shown that people with sleep disorders have more muscle imbalances and the prevalence of myofascial pains in these people is much higher than those who are able to get quality sleep.

Insomnia is a problem in which a person is unable to sleep. It can be due to emotional, physical, environmental, social, or mental factors, but the ultimate result of insomnia is myofascial pains in the neck, head, and back muscles. These people are always lethargic and possess very low strength in muscles. Moreover, postural imbalances in these people are also very common, which are the common causes of myofascial pain syndrome.

Hypersomnia refers to a state in which a person has to sleep more than the hours normally required. Sleeping more than required is also detrimental to health, as it poses severe strains on muscles leading to myofascial pains. In many studies, it is clearly found that people who sleep more than 8 hours are lethargic and possess myofascial pains, especially after waking up.

Poor sleeping posture is also the main reason behind sleep-associated myofascial pains. Many people complain that their pain gets worse when they wake up after sleep. The reason is prolonged pressure on affected muscles during sleep. Moreover, pain receptors are maximally active after sleep.

3. Depression, Anxieties, Fears and Panic Attacks

According to the current definition by The World Health Organization (WHO) health is a state of having optimal psychological, physical, emotional, and mental well-being.

However, they are trying to create their own definition of health, because no one can remain physically, mentally, psychologically, and emotionally well at a constant. There are times when we feel really depressed and down. People with a traumatic past are more prone to depressive disorders. Depression is a syndrome rather than a disease. Low mood for a prolonged period of time, along with symptoms of sleeplessness, anxieties, loneliness, and physical pains, is the true definition of depression. It is evident that people with depressive disorders are very prone to myofascial pain syndrome.

Apart from the mental impacts of anxieties and depression, physical symptoms are very common as well, and the most prevalent physical symptom of depression and anxieties is myofascial pain syndrome. The muscles present around the neck and cranial region are most involved, and it can be trigger points in these muscles or muscle spasms, which can lead to myofascial pain syndromes. Another common muscle involved is the trapezius.

People with chronic depressive disorders often say that they feel heaviness in the head and neck, which is actually the involuntary tightness in these muscles because of stress. In the next portion of this book, we will discuss how to manage stress-related myofascial pain syndromes, but it is very important to mention here that depressions and anxieties are the leading causes of myofascial pain syndromes in all genders and age groups. However, females are affected the most because of the severe prevalence of these disorders in females.

Anxiety is a state which triggers the fight or flight response in our body. Shivering in the body, dilation of the pupils, sweating, uncontrolled tightness in head and neck muscles, and stress can lead to myofascial pain syndrome in patients with chronic anxieties. Patients with social anxieties are most prone to myofascial pain because the prevalence of trigger points in the head and neck muscles are very high in these patients. Anxious people show involuntary tightness in the neck and head muscles because it is their protective response. It is also referred to as a protective posture, which is the characteristic posture of anxious people. The prevalence of fibromyalgia and arthritis-related myofascial pains are also very high in anxious and depressed patients.

Panic disorder refers to a state in which a person feels sudden and extreme fear. The people often exhibit severe stress in these panic situations, and most of them tend to perform abrupt movements such as running, hiding, or involuntary moments of arms and legs. These movements are not well controlled, and sudden contractions in muscles lead to severe muscle spasms and trigger points. Fascia is a loose covering over our muscles, and most of the time, fascia gets tangled in these poorly controlled movements, leading to dull pain in the arms, legs, head, or back depending upon the fascia involved.

People with more severe mental disturbances show severe signs of myofascial pains because of the increased risks of falls, aggressive responses, and protective postures. It is essential to spread awareness of myofascial pain syndrome and its association with these psycho-emotional illnesses, which are damaging hundreds and thousands of lives around the globe.

4. Female Gender and Pregnancies

The most prevalent risk factor of myofascial pains, which cannot be controlled, is the female gender. The body of the female is naturally very prone to muscle weaknesses, imbalances, myofascial trigger points, fibromyalgia, nerve entrapment, and arthritis. All these factors are prevalent causes of myofascial pain syndromes, which make females the real victims of myofascial pain. Researches have shown that 1 in 2 females are suffering from myofascial pain syndrome and the most affected females fall between 17-45 years old.

Pregnancy comes with a lot of complications in the female body, and the prevalence of myofascial pains is very high among pregnant females. As soon as a female is pregnant, many important changes begin to happen in the female body. Her pelvis becomes broader, muscles become weak, and muscle imbalances are very common because of rapid changes in posture.

Remember the swayback posture I discussed previously. This, along with lower cross syndrome, are common in pregnancy. Moreover, water accumulation in the body of females is another risk factor associated with fascial distortion and nerve entrapments because the compartments of the female body become filled with extra water content (called compartmental syndromes).

This condition of excessive fluid accumulation is called edema, which causes severe compression on the nerves exiting from muscles, and associated fascia around these nerves get tangled, leading to severe episodes of myofascial pains, especially at night. The ligaments, which are anchors to our joints and tendons, and are attachment sites of muscles, also become very weak in pregnancy. This causes excessive pressure on the muscles and fascia, leading to myofascial pain syndrome. I want to clarify the syndrome word again because you will find it everywhere in this book. A syndrome is the cluster of diseases that come together because these diseases are closely associated with each other.

The sources of these diseases can be the same, and thus the combined presence of all these illnesses is called a syndrome. Myofascial pains often present in the forms of syndromes rather than a disease because various issues are combined in this problem. A person often has severe muscle spasms, trigger points, fascial distortions, arthritis, and muscle imbalances at the same time, and all these issues fall under the umbrella of myofascial pain syndrome.

Another common risk factor associated with the female gender is the high prevalence of stress, depression, and anxieties in females, leading to myofascial pain syndrome. Studies have confirmed that the presence of myofascial pain syndrome, specifically in the female genders, has handicapped millions of females around the world.

Anorexia nervosa is a disease in which one restricts their calorie intake to a very dangerous level. This leads to severe malnutrition in these people, and thus the muscles don't get enough fuel to keep working in a proper manner. This condition leads to severe muscle weakness and extreme imbalances in the body, leading to severe episodes of myofascial pain syndrome. Statistically, females are more likely to suffer from anorexia nervosa.

Bulimia nervosa is a condition in which the sufferer binge eats and then induces vomiting to avoid weight loss. This induced vomiting causes severe strain on the neck and back muscles as well as the muscles of the back and abdomen being severely compromised because of repetitive induced vomiting. All these factors lead to myofascial pain syndrome in these people. The prevalence of fascial distortion is more common in bulimia nervosa. Statistically, females are more likely to suffer from Bulimia.

The use of contraceptive pills can cause severe weakness in the body as well as hormonal disturbances, and it can also compromise the proper functioning of the female body, which can lead to myofascial pain syndromes. Menstruation is a normal and physiological process of the female body that continues until menopause. Menstruation causes severe wear and tear in the vaginal walls, and this leads to sharp pain in the lower abdomen and back.

Some females experience unbearable pain during their periods, and these females are most prone to myofascial pains in the lower abdomen and low back areas. In some instances, myofascial pains in the legs are also evident during menstruation. You may experience dull, deep, and aching pain in and around your genital area, which is hard to explain and nearly impossible to locate. This is because of tangled or distorted pelvic fascia, which can be affected during menstruation, pregnancy, or sexual activities. Female pelvic organs are less protected compared to male organs, which causes an additional threat to these structures. The pelvic fascia covers these organs, which is not a very strong structure, and it can get distorted even in simple movements.

So, it is advised that females be very cautious about their health. Proper diet, high-intensity exercise, amazing flexibility, and peace of mind are the most important shields against myofascial pain syndrome in females. I will discuss this more in the treatment sections.

5. Rheumatoid Arthritis and Osteo Arthritis

Arthritis is a term that refers to the pain and swelling in a joint. A joint is a structure of our body that is made up of two or more bones that join each other in a capsule to make movements possible. Shoulder and hip joints are the most dynamic joints of the body. Some joints, such as hip and knee joints, bear most of the weight of the body while standing.

Osteoarthritis refers to the pain and swelling in weight-bearing joints. In this illness, the space between the bones of a weight-bearing joint gets compromised, leading to wear and tear of the surfaces of these bones. Osteoarthritis is a disease of the elderly population. It often involves the population of 50-70-year-olds, but thanks to the digital era, this disease is making its way to the early 30s as well. Females are mostly affected; however, the prevalence of this disease among males is also very high.

The reason to mention osteoarthritis here is its association with myofascial pain syndrome. In knee osteoarthritis, there is a severe compromise in thigh and calf muscles, and patients often experience severe myofascial pain in the calf, behind the thigh, or above the knee joint because of severe trigger points and muscle spasms. The reason for this myofascial pain in the associated joint is abnormal loading. In knee osteoarthritis, there is abnormal loading on joints, and most of the work has to be done by muscles, which get weaker over time, leading to myofascial pain and trigger points. Osteoarthritis of the hips is associated with severe myofascial pain in the lower back and hip muscles. Fascial distortion around the hip joint is very common in osteoarthritis of the hip.

Another similar condition is rheumatoid arthritis. Rheumatoid arthritis affects non-weight bearing joints, and it is not a specific disease of the elderly population. In rheumatoid arthritis, the autoimmunity of the human body affects its own joints, muscles, and organs, leading to pain and swelling in the finger, wrist, elbow, shoulder, hip, knee, and ankle joints. Neck and back muscles are also involved. Moreover, it can damage organs such as kidneys, liver, pancreas, etc. Depending upon the type and severity of rheumatoid arthritis, myofascial pains can be experienced in nearly every area of the body, but the most affected areas are the upper extremities. Myofascial pains are very common in the wrist and elbow because joint swelling in these areas causes abnormal strain on the associated muscles. Moreover, autoimmunity damages the muscles of these areas more frequently.

In rheumatoid arthritis, the muscles of the neck and back are also severely affected. If you are a patient of rheumatoid arthritis, you may have felt episodic pain in your low back and neck area, as well as around the elbow. This pain is different than joint pain because it's poorly localized, traveling, and dull. Distorted fascial structures in these areas cause a strange type of pain. The biggest problem with myofascial pains is that it is hard to identify the source and location of the pain. If you know the mechanism behind the pain, the diagnosis will be very easy and accurate, but it takes time and proper guidance to know your own myofascial pain.

6. Spinal Disc Issues

The spine is a very dynamic skeletal structure of the body that allows forward, backward, sidewise, and rotational movements. Similarly, there are muscles and fascia distributed in all these directions to make these movements possible. If the fascia around a specific spinal segment gets distorted, it can severely compromise the proper movement of that specific segment of our spine. Similarly, if a jerky or abrupt movement is performed at the spine and in a specific direction, that can lead to severe tangling and distortion of fascia in that particular direction. So, this delicate and sensitive relationship between different spinal structures makes it very prone to myofascial pains and injuries.

The spine is further divided into the cervical spine, which is actually our neck, thoracic spine, or upper and middle back, as well as the lower back, which is called the lumbar spine. The irony of myofascial pain syndrome is, it involves every segment of our spine equally, and the myofascial pain around these areas is considered one of the most painful experiences based on a pain intensity survey. Many muscles are present around our spine, and these muscles are very prone to trigger points, tender points, and spasms because they are postural in nature.

Postural muscles are those that don't have enough strength to produce a lot of forceful contractions, but these muscles are eligible to hold our bodies against gravity for a longer period of time. When a person adopts a faulty posture habitually, or he/she performs a poorly coordinated movement at the spine, these muscles, and fascia around them can be hurt, leading to mild to severe myofascial pains.

Another issue that leads to myofascial pains around the spine is the spinal disc issue. The spine is made up of 33 vertebras, and most of them have discs between two adjacent vertebras. The function of these discs is to control the movements of the spine and shock absorption during the loading phases. However, these discs are prone to injuries as well and an injured or prolapsed disc can compress the exiting nerves at that particular spinal segment.

The most prevalent spinal disc issue is sciatica, which is characterized as severe pain in one or both legs starting from the lower back to the sole of the feet. This is because of the compression of the sciatic nerve by bulged discs in the lumbar spine. Sciatic pain is the true example of myofascial pain syndrome because it is often associated with multiple trigger points and muscle tightness in the hip, buttock, back, thigh, and calf muscles. Even in a false form of sciatica, there is no compression on the sciatic nerve in the lumbar spine, but the whole leg and buttock are still hurting because of myofascial trigger points in various muscles of the leg.

Spinal disc bulge in the cervical spine causes severe myofascial pains in the upper extremities. Have you experienced pain that runs from the neck to your fingers and numbness in your arm and elbow as well as in the first three fingers? This pain is because of C5 nerve compression in the cervical spine. This compression leads to very painful trigger points in the trapezius muscle, bicep, deltoid, and forearm muscles. Moreover, the severe pain in these areas is also because the fascia around the arm and neck gets distorted, leading to very severe pain in the upper extremity. In many instances, the patient fails to lift his arm above the head, and his sleep is severely compromised because he cannot bear the pain after lying on the affected side. The worst part of this myofascial pain is the difficulty of diagnosing it, and it is often confused with other disorders.

7. Fibrosis Scarring and Immobilization

Fibrosis, as a process, is less linear than scarring, which typically occurs step by step in a sequence. Fibrosis usually involves the connective tissues and structures of an entire region. The process of fibrosis can occur in at least two distinct fashions. The first may be associated with the imbalance of collagen production from a nearby traumatic site. Studies have indicated that the process of fibrosis is accelerated during wound repair and that neighboring tissue can become involved. Doctors have noticed fibrosis can occur anywhere in the body, i.e. from top to toe, as well as progressively through tissue distant from the traumatized area.

Cell atrophy is yet another condition where connective tissue can be altered negatively, creating an avenue for potential injury. Secondary to stress response, metabolic activities can decrease or cease altogether. Once started in this cycle, e.g. from immobilization, energy production decreases along with other functions. This leads to degeneration and increased vulnerability to injury.

One of the many frustrations of immobilization is myofascial pains, because the muscles and fascia lose their extensibility, leading to tightness, adhesions, and trigger points. Immobilization occurs in both static and dynamic situations. The typical type of immobilization is a static form that involves braces, casts, wraps, traction, fusion, etc. Other immobilizations that occur are those secondary to minor traumas, which can lead to protective muscle spasm or infections and further lead to adhesions.

Still, another form of immobilization could be classified as progressive in nature, such as bone spurring in osteoarthritis or the immobility noted secondary to fibromyalgia. At some level, with all these examples, there exists a condition where either internal or external fixation of body parts occurs. It is important to manage immobilization but having active rest, i.e. moving the associated areas more often to avoid adhesions. It has been noted that, at least at times, atrophy is far more detrimental to the remobilization of tissues than scarring.

8. Myofascial Trigger Points

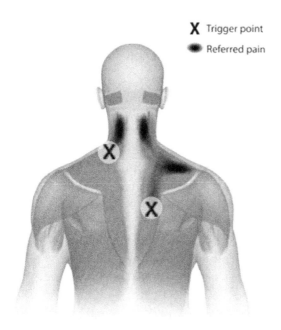

Trigger points are tight bands in muscles that have a characteristic knot in the middle. Due to local trauma to the muscle as a result of overuse, overstretching, deconditioning, injury or illness, trigger points may form in a small number of muscle fibers in a larger muscle or muscle bundle. There are hundreds of potential trigger points in human muscles, and they reportedly show up in the same places in every person. In an active trigger point, pain can either be local or felt in another location, called referred pain.

Latent trigger points are those that are perceived as a painful knot only after palpation. Any muscle can develop an individual trigger point or multiple points. The neck and shoulders, lower back and buttocks, middle back, thighs, and calves are the most prone areas for developing myofascial trigger points.

Latent and active trigger points (TRPs) can lead to poor muscle coordination and balance. Many people call active and latent trigger points "ouch" points, whereby just pressing on the point elicits pain (people with fibromyalgia understand this all too well). When trigger points are present in muscles, there's often pain and weakness in the associated structures. There are various theories associated with trigger points, but the most acceptable theory is hyper irritation theory, which suggests that the trigger points cause over-stimulation of the muscle, leading to the activation of pain in associated nerves.

Today, treatment of trigger points is administered by massage therapists, physical therapists, osteopathic physicians, occupational therapists, myotherapists, athletic trainers, chiropractors, and acupressure practitioners. Practitioners claim to have identified reliable referred pain patterns that associate pain in one location with trigger points elsewhere. The compression of a trigger point may elicit local tenderness, referred pain, or local twitch response.

There are also subtle trigger points that are present throughout the course of a nerve. These trigger points are not present at the actual area of source pain, and thus they are very confusing in nature.

Myofascial trigger points are "hot spots" in the fascia that irritate nearby muscle cells, causing them to contract. Trigger points often develop after an injury, mechanical stress, or repetitive micro trauma—all conditions under which the fascia becomes "sticky". This combination of contracted muscle cells and sticky fascia creates a taut, painful lump or band. When the fascia is already contracted and irritable, it is very easy to develop these hot spots, and trigger points are quite common in fibromyalgia. One study found an average of twelve of these hot spots in subjects with fibromyalgia, with healthy controls having one or none.

Focusing on treating those trigger points can reduce local muscle pain. The most effective treatments involve physically disrupting the tissue by stretching, massage, or insertion of a needle into the muscle.

Trigger point injections—inserting needles with a numbing medicine—that break up these tissue knots have been shown to be helpful in fibromyalgia. One study found reduced muscle pain compared to placebo injections that were done near, but not into, trigger points. Another showed reduced pain and increased range of motion in fibromyalgia patients after trigger point injection. It is important to note that some fibromyalgia patients have lots of trigger points, too many actually, to be able to treat them with trigger point injections.

Some physical therapists also offer dry needling, the use of needles alone to break up the trigger point. It has also been shown to be effective, but the addition of numbing medicines reduces the intensity and duration of post-injection soreness.

Focused, intense finger pressure and some other massage techniques can also undo a contraction knot. A technique called "spray and stretch" puts a numbing medication on the skin and then performs intense stretching to break up a trigger point.

Whatever method you choose, softening the tight and knotted areas of fascia can dramatically reduce muscle pain.

9. Fibromyalgia and Tender Points

Fibromyalgia is known as some very specific but episodic pains and early fatigue because the muscles are sore, and there are characteristic knots in several areas of the body. These knots are primarily present in muscles, but different from trigger points.

Trigger points are hyperirritable spots that are not as big as the tender points are. A characteristic tender point can be 3-5cm in diameter and extremely painful when pressed or irritated.

Tender points are formed when a muscle is pushed beyond its limits and because fibromyalgia causes severe fatigue in the body. Both the tender points and the mother condition, fibromyalgia, is causing a severe compromise in the quality of life of hundreds and thousands of patients.

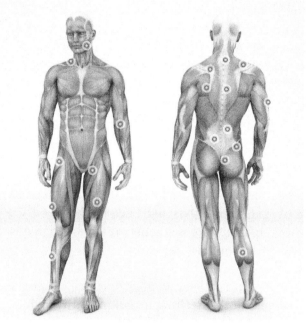

Fibromyalgia is a leading cause of myofascial pain syndrome because it is a long-term condition, and there is no single effective remedy to cure the disease completely. The best way to avoid myofascial pain in fibromyalgia patients is to know the limits of a muscle. The most effective treatment approaches are rest, icing, heating, stretching, foam rolling, massage, and electrotherapy, which will be discussed in the next sections of this book.

Fibromyalgia is extremely common, affecting at least 3 percent of the population in the United States (Lawrence 1998; White 1999). It doesn't discriminate by socioeconomic class: my patients include fast-food workers, lawyers, custodians, school district superintendents, zookeepers, and teachers. While it predominantly affects women, many more men, especially combat veterans, have been diagnosed in recent years.

Most patients first seek medical guidance for persistent pain or fatigue, but they may also experience irritable bowel and bladder symptoms, low blood pressure, poor balance, dizziness on standing, headaches, sensitivity to loud noises and numbness or tingling in hands or feet. All of these symptoms can be tied in one way or another to dysfunction in the stress response.

Given the prevalence of fibromyalgia and how much research has now been done, it seems like it should be easy for health care providers to diagnose, doesn't it? Unfortunately, that's not the case because there are no accepted imaging or blood tests that can confirm a diagnosis. Complicating matters, its symptoms are not unique; similar problems can be caused by anemia, hypothyroidism, and chronic fatigue syndrome. If you see your doctor for fatigue or muscle pain, the workup usually starts with lab tests for thyroid function, red blood cell count, and inflammation in the blood as she tries to rule out other potential causes. Standard laboratory tests come back *normal* in fibromyalgia, so it is considered a diagnosis of exclusion, given only after no other sources of muscle pain and fatigue have been found.

Fibromyalgia Is a Clinical Diagnosis
The lack of lab abnormalities associated with fibromyalgia and the fact that sufferers don't "look sick" have contributed to the controversy surrounding this illness. Technically, fibromyalgia is not even considered a disease; it is still referred to in the medical literature as a *syndrome:* a collection of signs, symptoms, and medical problems that tend to occur together but are not related to a specific, identifiable cause. A *disease,* meanwhile, has a specific cause or causes and recognizable signs and symptoms. As you will learn, I do feel that there is a specific cause for fibromyalgia and thus refer to it as a disease or illness throughout this book.

To ease the difficulty of diagnosing fibromyalgia, in 1990, a group of rheumatologists created a set of diagnostic criteria for doctors and researchers (Wolfe 1990). Patients with fibromyalgia have "widespread pain in multiple connective tissue areas" (Mease 2011), and through trial and error, these rheumatologists found that most patients were very tender in eighteen specific points in the muscles. These muscles were present at the flank area, below the knees, in thighs, buttock and in the neck and over the second ribs, near the breastbone. To be diagnosed with fibromyalgia, you need a history of diffuse musculoskeletal pain and tenderness on palpation (applied pressure) in eleven of those eighteen points.

Fibromyalgia Versus Chronic Fatigue Syndrome
As a general rule for CFS, patients are very tired all day long but don't necessarily have physical pains. Fibro patients always have pain AND are often very tired too. Doctors and patients alike are confused by the similarities between chronic fatigue syndrome (CFS) and fibromyalgia (FM).

Both are poorly understood conditions that are characterized by fatigue and primarily affect women. Complicating matters further, the two terms are often used interchangeably or lumped together and treated as if they were the same disease, under the banner of "FM/CFS". Many of my patients think they must have chronic fatigue syndrome because they feel fatigued all the time, and this is a common misperception.

But there are actually very specific criteria for CFS—it has unique symptoms, different triggers (for example, the fatigue stems from a dysfunctional immune system), and responds to different treatments. Most CFS patients describe a sudden onset of symptoms, often after a flu-like illness, suggesting that it may be triggered by an infection. For the past thirty years, researchers have theorized that it is caused by a viral infection because of certain tell-tale changes seen in the blood and immune cells of CFS patients.
However, no one has been able to identify a specific instigating virus, so it is now thought that a few different types of viral infections may trigger the immune system to go haywire. It is this overactive immune response, not a viral infection, that leads to fatigue, low-grade fevers, sore throat, and swollen lymph nodes. Fibromyalgia, on the other hand, usually has a gradual onset and is not associated with fevers, sore throats, or lymph node swelling.

Myofascial release is a manual therapy that reduces tension in the fascia, the connective tissue around muscles. You will learn more about using this therapy to reduce fibromyalgia pain, but it also induces a relaxation response in the body.

Fascia contains many fight-or-flight nerve endings, and gentle sustained pressure of myofascial release calms them and lowers their activity (Tanaka 1977). A study found reduced signals from fight-or-flight nerves for twenty-four hours after this therapy was applied to the pelvic fascia (Cottingham 1988). Fascial stretching sends a "calm down" message through the fight-or-flight nerves back up to the brain stem, turning down fight-or-flight and turning up rest-and-digest, with lingering relaxation effects. You can also self-administer myofascial release.

10.Injuries and Accidents

All of us will experience a variety of accidents and injuries during our lives, from childhood through to old age. You may immediately have thought of something, such as a car crash, breaking a leg, or similar. A major trauma will usually be remembered long after the event and can have long-lasting effects. These effects may be apparent in the weeks and months after an accident, but they can also emerge years later, having been carried in the fascia long after superficial healing takes place, whether or not you have obvious scars.

Even those everyday minor incidents, such as bumping into a kitchen cupboard, missing your footing as you step off a curb, or stubbing your toe, can create fascial injuries that are communicated deeper into the body. What may soon be forgotten by the conscious mind stays with us and can have consequences later in life.

Both major and minor accidents are relatively high impact compared with other forms of injury to the fascia, and both are likely to cause snagging and tearing. These snags and tears, and the healing processes that take place around them, create imbalances and fresh lines of tension within the body that pull on surrounding areas, causing physical and other problems.

For example, if you are involved in a car accident, you may experience whiplash, a soft tissue injury that occurs when your head is suddenly jolted forward and then back. Whiplash damages the fascia in your neck and shoulders. As more collagen fibers are created to patch and strengthen the tears, restrictions develop. These restrictions create stiffness that limits movement, and abnormal tensions result in further issues. For one person, the consequence could be headaches, and for another, it might be lower back pain.

There is another aspect of high-impact fascial injury, and that relates to energy. Again, taking the example of a car crash, in addition to creating visual and other memories, the high impact of the event causes energy to become stuck in the fascia in the form of tissue memory, which then becomes associated with emotion. The immediate pain of an accident and unresolved damage to the fascia can lead to chronic pain.

How well our fascia heals after an accident depends partly on how healthy it was to start with and partly on how we treat it afterward. That is why an understanding of fascial anatomy and the energetic properties of fascia is so important in treatment and self-help after accidents.

11.Overuse of Muscles

As fluid beings, we are designed to move and to use our bodies. However, as our world has become more advanced, systems, machines, and gadgets have been invented that have changed our lifestyles and how we move.

Overuse and underuse are related and growing problems arising from our modern lifestyles, including work and leisure. Both cause fascial injuries.

Most people actually subject their bodies to a powerful combination of underuse and overuse that can almost be characterized as abuse.

There is barely a client I see who does not, in some way, attribute the physical (and mental) stress they feel and the problems they experience to the work they do. Similarly, very few see exercise as a problem. For some of us, work is the only physical activity we do. If we did not work, we would be in a worse state. For others, the problem is the intensity with which we pursue our leisure activities, whether in the gym or with the X-box.

The following examples will be recognizable to many, but it is important not to fall for stereotypes. Damaging overuse can happen in everyday situations if our job demands that we do any limited action repeatedly for long periods. Equally, underuse can be just as damaging. And we may do more damage to ourselves outside work than in it.

The important thing is to start to gain an understanding of the demands that any activity or inactivity makes on our fascia.

12. Work and Ergonomics

According to the World Health Organization, most of us will spend at least one-third of our life at work, and work is a dangerous place to be! Some of us work in arduous physical industries where better health and safety is needed to reduce the risk of accident, while others are at risk of "ergonomic injuries" that demand better awareness of occupational health.

Ergonomic injuries affect those of us who do manual work and those of us who work in an office. In both contexts, our work has become more specialized, or the need to move has been reduced. This process has been affecting ever greater numbers of people since the early days of the industrial revolution.

Previously, many traditional forms of manual labor required great strength and flexibility. People were required to move their bodies in different directions continually and with varying degrees of force, as jobs became more mechanized, this need lessened. In factories, production lines developed. These again reduced the need to move, because now the work came to you, and divided previously broad jobs into ever smaller, specialized tasks requiring a reduced repertoire of movement. We have now reached the stage where robots may do the production line work while we sit in a control room, staring at a computer screen.

In offices, the process has been similar. In the typing pools of the 1950s and 1960s, the women (as it generally was) who operated manual typewriters worked in a highly organized environment but still had a certain degree of movement in their work. They needed to use force to press the typewriter keys and shoulder movements to operate the carriage return at the end of every line. As they finished each typed sheet, the paper would need to be changed, and this provided an opportunity to roll and stretch their shoulders. Every so often, they would get up to deliver their work to a central collection point and to pick up more.

In modern offices, we now operate ever decreasing sizes of keyboards that require minimal movement of our hands and fingers. We hunch over for hours on end, stuck in one position, staring at our computer screen. The need to get up and physically move to talk to colleagues has been replaced by email and instant messaging.

All of this has an effect on our fascia. For as long as we keep moving, our fascia remains fluid, but if we stay in one position for more than 2 minutes (yes, *2 minutes!*), our body thinks we want to make a permanent change and starts to lay down new fascia to help with this. At this stage, this new fascia is a light fuzzy tissue, a bit like fluff or candy floss. If you move normally after a few minutes, this candy floss will melt away and be reabsorbed. But time spent stuck in one position, hour after hour, day after day, for months and years creates more and more layers of fascia which no longer stay light and fuzzy. The layers start to stick together like Velcro and harden, eventually becoming like plywood.

This is underuse in action. We are not moving enough to keep our body mobile. The impact of this is far-reaching. Over time our muscles become less able to stretch and may even start to calcify (turn to bone), bones become harder and more brittle, nerves, blood vessels, and organs are literally squeezed to the point that they no longer function properly.

At the same time as underuse, our work situations often create overuse of specific parts of the body. For example, working at a computer for many hours, day in day out, involves chronic overuse of the muscles and fascia in our forearms and hands. None of these muscles are particularly big, which means it does not take much to tire them. However, if we keep typing and using our mouse, we overuse these muscles and irritate them to the point of damage, as the fascia that surrounds them becomes stuck into one big irritating lump of tissue.

The need for our fascia to remain fluid and free-moving to shift and accommodate our organs, will help you to appreciate why the underuse and overuse exemplified by the western "sitting epidemic" have become a major issue resulting in all sorts of problems, including digestive and respiratory ones.

PART 3) Self Treatments at Home

So, we have covered almost all of the risk factors and causes of myofascial pain syndrome. Remember, knowing the cause is 50% of the treatment because the notorious myofascial pain is hard to diagnose. I suffered half of my life.

Medicines caused severe compromise on my digestive health, and I was frustrated because I never felt relief. As soon as I started learning about myofascial pain, I immediately turned my focus on knowing the cause rather than rushing towards the treatment.

You can have rheumatoid arthritis, or you maybe have fibromyalgia; trigger points can limit your daily activities, or your posture is really bad. Whatever the cause is, you have to find it and adjust it. Your pain will not automatically go away but remember, treat the cause, do not treat the symptom. Pain is a symptom, not a cause.

In this portion of the book, I will discuss some really effective treatments of myofascial pain, but the best thing is, you can do all these remedies on your own because I intended to write this book as a self-management guide for myofascial pain.

The following are the main self-treatment strategies for myofascial pain syndrome, and I will explain each of them:
o   Management with your hands
o   Management with foam rolls
o   Management with the Thera Cane
o   Management with balls
o   Management with stretching
o   Management with massage
o   Management with reflexology
o   Management with heating
o   Management with icing (Cryotherapy)
o   Management with electrotherapy devices

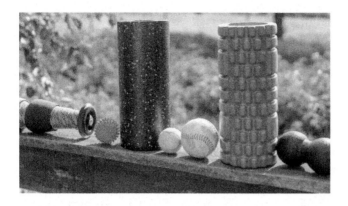

Foam rollers and balls are the most commonly used tools to release muscle knots at home, but there are other tools available. Simply search for "tools for myofascial release". Every person is different, and one tool might work for one person whilst not for the other.

Other myofascial release treatments are acupuncture and dry needling but of course, you can't do these yourself, therefore I will not cover these in detail.

Yoga is also very effective to treat fascia problems. Do certain yoga poses that treat the area where you feel pain. It is a very broad subject and thus is a whole book of its own! You can find a lot of information about this in yoga books, online and on YouTube.

Yin Yoga (holding poses for a long time; from 2 to 5 minutes) is especially good for myofascial release. Restorative Yoga and Micro Yoga are good too.

With yoga: always start with holding a pose for 20 to 30 seconds and gradually increase the time you hold. For some people, holding for too long can actually make things worse, so be careful.

Research has shown that stretching, relaxation, meditation, trigger point treatments, and biofeedback techniques ease muscle tension that contributes to pain. Regular stretching is useful to release muscle tension and lengthen shortened muscles, decreasing pain. Massage is most people's favorite because it can reduce anxiety, contributing to reducing muscle tension. Massage can also increase blood flow to an area, which may hasten to heal. Performing simple self-myofascial release moves daily with the foam roller can keep muscles fluid, prevent future issues, and offer many other benefits.

Osteopathy and myofascial pain
Osteopathic techniques have been used the early 1800s to treat myofascial pains. Osteopaths often use the energy of involved muscles to treat the tightness or painful knots in muscles. These techniques are called muscle energy techniques. Most of these osteopathic techniques involve active contractions of muscles along with active or passive muscle stretching (resistive stretch). Covering osteopathic techniques here is beyond the scope of this self-help book.

However, it is a great idea to consult an experienced DO (doctor of osteopathy) for your myofascial pains before treating your muscles and fascia through self-release techniques.

1. How does it work and what will you achieve?
Firstly, it is important to visit your doctor to eliminate any other muscle diseases or medical conditions before you start myofascial release at home.

Find your muscle knots
To find muscle knots, as they don't always give you pain, you can simple "feel" your body. Literally, with your hands, rub everywhere over your body and you might feel little bumps or aches whilst you are doing these. Chances are high these are muscle knots or trigger points.

Say you feel an ache in your upper left thigh. You can lie on a foam roller and roll up and down on your upper thigh. Roll steady and slowly. When you feel a little knot, which will feel like a little bump, keep the pressure on that for a few seconds, and then roll up and down again. Come back to the knot and you can often simply just feel an "aha" moment, where your body will just "sink" into the knot and you can feel the release. This means you have successfully done a myofascial release.

The same principle applies when using balls for releases.

Another way to find where your fascia is stuck is to do stretches.

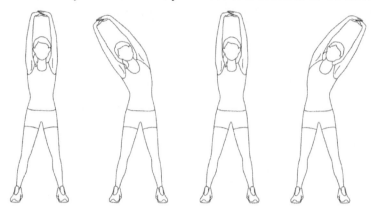

For example, do a side stretch as shown on the picture above and you might feel certain areas are pretty tight or you feel some muscles pulling. Roll on a foam roller or a ball on these tight areas and do the stretch again. You might be surprised, and the tight area might now feel completely normal. That's how easy release can be.

The bottom line is that with myofascial treatment at home you can get rid of the muscle knots in the areas where you feel pain. By releasing the knots, your muscles can function optimally again, and your pain will go. After all, the muscle was shortened because of the muscle knot, so you need to stretch the muscle after release.

Remember, whichever tool you use for releasing, always stretch afterwards e.g. if you have released a knot in your arm, stretch your arm for 10 to 20 seconds afterwards.

Fascia loves heat
Fascia loves heat and especially damp heat. Sometimes after a release you might experience some aches. These are some methods you can use to ease the pain:
- A warm bath with Epsom salt
- A warm bath with |Magnesium flakes
- A heated blanket
- Sit in the sun
- A sauna
- A steam room

The pain is often not the area to treat

Very often, the area where you feel the pain is NOT the area that you need to treat. This is due to the trigger points, which we have discussed previously.

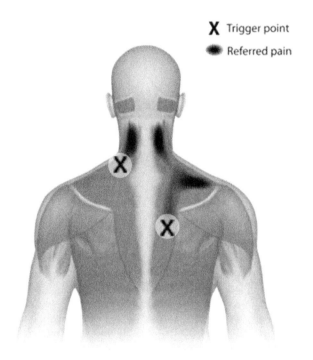

Simply explained: often the area where you feel the pain (see referred pain on the drawing above) is NOT the area to treat with a myofascial release tool. The area to use the tool is actually where the "X" is on the drawing. If you would treat the referred pain area, you wouldn't actually solve the pain problem as the pain problem or trigger point is the "X".

Visit www.triggerpoints.net to find where your pain areas and trigger points are. This is a really good website to help you with myofascial release. Should this website no longer be live when you read this book, just search for "trigger points and referred pain".

For example, the trigger point in the neck muscles can trigger headaches, and the trigger point in the buttocks can trigger sciatica (pain that can be in the whole leg). Active trigger points are those which cause myofascial pain even without stimulation.

Latent trigger points are those which cause pain only when they are pressed. Trigger points can also be present in a complete myofascial sling. Their pain runs in specific patterns, but after identification, these tight knots can easily be treated with the help of well-planned and skilled self-treatments.

Important warnings
Releasing a knot or rolling on a knot should be a "good pain" instead of real pain. Stop immediately, with whatever treatment discussed in this book, if you feel real pain. You will soon learn the difference between muscle knot pain and real pain.

You must be very careful when doing self-treatment on these areas, as they contain a lot of muscles and nerves. Pushing too hard for too long can actually create nerve and/or muscle damage in:
- Back of your knees
- Your sit bone or coccyx bone.
- Your pelvic area

Also be careful when rolling on your spine. Never roll too hard for too long. Furthermore, never roll over a bone.

As a general rule, leave 24 hours between treatments after you have done a release, so the muscles have time to adjust. If you have released several muscle knots in one sitting, it is better not to do any exercises or fitness training for 24 to 48 hours.

2. Management With Your Hands
There is a difference between fascia release and muscle knot release. You can do fascia release without actually pushing any knots.

Say, for example, you have a dull and minor ache in your upper left thigh. To release the fascia: put your left hand just above your left knee and your right hand on your right side of that upper thigh. **Very slowly** pull the skin down with your left hand and up with your right hand. Hold this for 30 to 60 seconds. Now you are pulling your fascia without touching a trigger point or a knot. Sometimes this small action can release tiny "wrinkles" in the fascia and pull it straight again. Your dull ache might disappear.

This action of "pulling" facia can be applied to any part of your body but, of course, keeping the warnings in mind explained in this book.

Releasing muscle knots is totally different. As explained above, you can just feel your body for muscle knots. Sometimes it is actually really simple to release with your hands. This is not possible for difficult-to-reach body parts and also not possible for "stubborn" muscle knots or knots that have been sitting in your body for years.

Simply push the trigger point with your finger or thumb for 10 to 30 seconds and often you can just feel the muscle knot melting away.

Although this might sound easy to do, it can become painful in your fingers or thumbs if you have a lot of knots and therefore have to use your fingers a lot. Luckily, there are tools available to help you and you can also strengthen your fingers and thumbs.

Instead of using your fingers, you can use tools to push on the muscle knots. The picture below shows a "knobble" (top left), the "original knobble" (bottom) and a massage roller ball (on the right). You can buy these tools on many online shops.

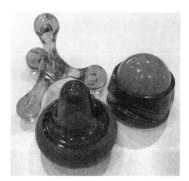

If you prefer to use your fingers or thumbs instead of tools, here is a picture of some strengthening products: hand grip and finger exerciser (on the left), rubber ring, elastic bands to stretch your fingers, and finger stretchers. You can buy these on many online shops.

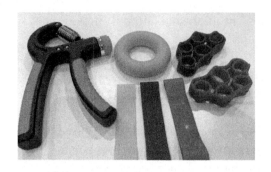

3. Management With Foam Rollers

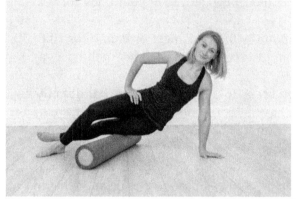

Too often, chronic poor posture and improper body mechanics, along with overtraining specific muscles, lead to increased muscle tension and muscle imbalances. Additionally, trauma to an area can also increased muscle tension, which often contributes to muscle spasms. Often, as a result of trauma to an area, a person develops "knots" or "trigger point discomfort."

If these dysfunctions aren't addressed properly, they can lead to reduced mobility and chronic problems. Performing myofascial techniques with the trigger point foam roller along with a systematic stretching routine can facilitate the break-up of these sticky adhesions.

The beauty of the programs in this book is that they can be done as stand-alone routines or performed in conjunction with your regular training regimen, either prior to or after a workout to relax tight muscles. In any case, they work to break up interwoven muscle fibers to improve blood flow into the muscles. The only requirement of the program is time on task and being in tune with your body's communication system.

How to manage trigger points using foam rolls
The concept behind self-myofascial release methods is to think of yourself as a world-class massage therapist. Good massage therapists don't say, "I'll spend five minutes on your legs and three minutes on your shoulders." Instead, they allow your body to provide them feedback via their hands of where to go and how hard to press. In a similar fashion, you should let your body tell you what it wants. Some days you'll need to spend more time on your upper back, while on other days, you'll want more time on your legs—just follow your body's suggestions.

We possess varying thresholds of discomfort, and each body part requires different amounts of pressure. Aim for what "hurts so good". Start with a light touch and move to deeper pressure. The legs are often very sensitive, whereas the back, buttocks, and shoulders often can tolerate more pressure.

 Exercise caution when performing any releases around the abdominal and neck regions or any area where you have any health issues. It's okay to press a tight spot until uncomfortable, and then back off. While some experts suggest holding a spot for long periods of time, this experience is not a test of your pain tolerance! Don't let anyone "should" you! Use your common sense.

To obtain optimal results, tune out external distractions and tune in to your internal communication. The most important thing is to relax when doing myofascial release with foam rollers or balls. The second most important is your breathing. The time you spend doing self-massage with the foam roller should be a mindful experience. If you stay mindful of your body's instructions, it will direct you where to place the roller, how much intensity you should place against your body, and how long to hold the position. Using the foam roller in combination with mindful breathing can aid in the outcome. Mindful breathing is an active awareness of the breathing process.

There's no absolute right way to perform each movement. Some days, significant pressure will feel fine, while on other days, the slightest pressure hurts. When doing self-massage, try to start at the proximal (top) parts of the body or limb. For example, start at the thigh and move toward the foot.

Mindful breathing

In mindful breathing, you will be aware of inhalation, exhalation, depth of breathing, and frequency of breathing. It helps in actively controlling the pain processes. Research has shown that breathing is directly related to the intensity of pain, and a mindful breathing pattern while performing myofascial release helps in the reduction of abnormal pain signals from affected muscles and fascia. Breathing is important, whichever method of release you choose. A suggested breathing plan is to inhale slowly, either through the nose or mouth fully, for a count of 4 to 6, and then exhale slowly through the lips (as if blowing out a candle) for a count of 8 to 12. If you inhale really deeply, your whole upper body will move up and down and this way pressure will come off and on the foam roller whilst you are lying on the roller. This up and down motion is extra good for releasing muscle knots.

Guidelines to using foam rolls

There are different types of foam rollers on the market. The differences are in the texture, length and thickness. The most important is the texture of the foam roller, which determines how hard the foam rollers are. These are the main types of floor foam rollers:

- Soft
- Medium
- Hard
- Very hard
- Spiky

There is no right or wrong here, it all depends on what your body likes. Generally speaking, soft rollers are more suitable for fibromyalgia patients.

Furthermore, there are also rollers that you can use with your hands as shown on the picture below. In this book, I will focus on floor rollers.

You can use foam rollers in short bouts of 30 seconds to 2 minutes. Rest for 2-3 minutes before reusing the foam rollers on affected muscles or fascia. You can have 3-5 sets of foam roller technique per day.

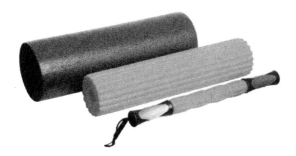

If you feel worse after a session, consider reducing the intensity and duration of the session. Remember that self-massage and myofascial-release sessions are not magical cures. If you're experiencing chronic pain, it's imperative that you ascertain the cause by seeking medical advice. Masking pain with a massage is no better than masking your pain with drugs or alcohol.

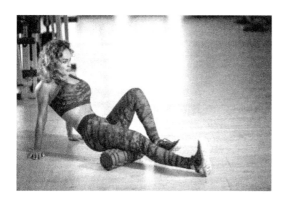

Usually you will roll the foam roller in the direction of your muscles. As shown on the above picture, by moving your body up and down, whilst leaning onto your arms, you will roll your leg over the roller. Find the sore spot and hold the roller there for a while, then roll up and down again.

The key to effective use of trigger point foam rollers lies in the following concepts:

- Understand how long and how much pressure to apply.
- Understand the expected outcomes of the program.
- Be relaxed and warm.
- Dress in clothes that allow you freedom of movement.
- Understand the interconnectedness of how tight hamstrings influence lower back pain. Learn which order of treatment is best for you. Generally, large muscle groups are followed by isolated muscles
- Focus on areas of tension, but don't go beyond mild discomfort. Benefits are not going to come if you're in pain, since pain causes tightness. You should feel better when you release it.
- Be patient; don't expect overnight results. You don't need to hold the position to the point of pain.
- While self-massage is generally considered safe, it's still wise to be cautious.
- Never massage an area where inflammation or swelling is present.
- Never massage a bony area.
- Never do too much too soon.
- Avoid any area that has been injured until cleared by your health provider.
- Speak to your health provider if you're pregnant or have osteoporosis.
- Seek medical advice if you're in poor health, in severe pain, and have a poor range of motion/flexibility.
- When lying on the foam roller, align your spine correctly. A correct lying posture causes minimum pressure on your spine by maintaining the natural curves of the spine.
- Don't focus on duration—use your body as a guide.
- No particular direction is right or wrong but most of the time good results are obtained by rolling in the directions of the muscles.

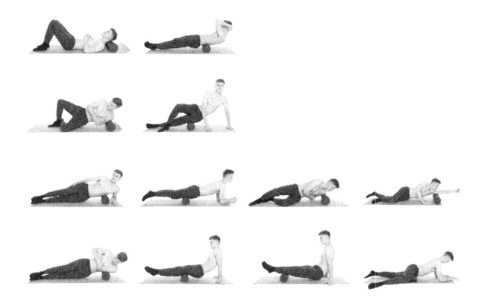

Trigger point foam rollers are a wonderful way to improve mobility and release tension while adding diversity to your standard exercise program. Just remember: if you allow too much time to elapse between sessions, the adhesions reform, and you have to start over. A little bit done regularly is far more beneficial than a lot done infrequently.

Some sample techniques

Mid-Back Release
Target: Mid-back

The Position: Lie on the roller so that it's under your spine from your tailbone to your neck. Knees should be flexed and place your feet flat pressing against the floor. Extend your arms out to the sides along the floor into a "T" position. Hold for 5 to 30 seconds. Breathe slowly and fully.

Modification: To challenge your core, reach your arms up to the ceiling. You can also straighten your legs to increase the pressure, as well as roll left and right.

Lower Back Expansion
Target: Lower back
Caution: if you have lumbar spine issues, you have to be cautious with this exercise.
The Position: Your back against the floor and knees should be flexed. Place the roller directly under your lower back. Gently press your lower back into the roller and hold for 5 to 30 seconds. Breathe slowly and deeply.

Hip Flexor Extender
Target: Lower back, hip flexors
Starting Position: Flex your knees and lie straight by pressing your back with floor and feet flat on the floor. Place the roller directly under your lower back.
Gently press your lower back into the roller and hold for 5 to 30 seconds. Breathe slowly and deeply. Then grab under your right thigh and gently pull your knee to your chest as you extend your left leg to the floor. Hold.
Switch legs.
Modification: If flexibility is an issue, lie on the roller from head to tailbone.

Total Calf Release
Target: Calves
This can be performed on one or both calves at the same time.
Starting Position: Sit with your legs extended, propping yourself up on your elbows and hands. Now, put the roller beneath the calf muscle near the knee.
Using your arms to move your legs, slowly roll the roller up and down the backs of your calves. Hold at tender locations as needed. Switch sides.
Modification: This can also be done while lying face up.
Variation: You can also turn your foot inward and outward to get the inside and outside of the calf.

Inner thigh Release
Target: Adductor muscles (inner thigh muscles).
Starting Position: Sit in a squat position and extend the leg to be treated. Place the foam roller beneath the extend leg (under inner

thigh muscles) and perform to and fro motions on the foam roller (move the inner thigh over foam roller).

Variation: You can use your hand to press the inner thigh on the foam roller. This is important when you want to treat deeper layers of inner thigh muscles.

Lateral thigh Release

Target: Abductor muscles (Muscles on the outer side of the thigh).
Starting Position: Lie down on your side. The thigh to be treated will be on the floor. Place a foam roller below the outer thigh muscles and simply move over the foam roller by pressing it between the outer thigh muscles and the ground.
Variation: You can use more pressure to treat the deeper layers of outer thigh muscles, but too much pressure can cause soreness.

4. Management With The Thera Cane

The Thera Cane is a long, tubular rod that has various extensions on it. One end of the Thera Cane is U-shaped, which is also called the treatment zone because it is mostly used to treat the areas which are harder to reach otherwise. The Thera Cane comes in various colors but these varying colors are just for appearance.

The extensions on the Thera Cane have circular balls, which are used to treat myofascial trigger points (muscle knots) and tender points. The lower end of the Thera Cane is a straight tube, which is also called "the holder." Below is a picture of a Thera Cane.

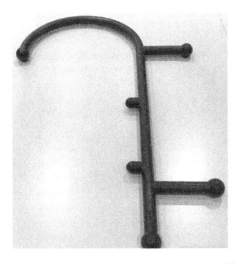

To use the Thera Cane for myofascial release, simply press the painful area with the head of the Thera Cane. It is important that you press the targeted area with enough pressure to feel the release beneath the head of the Thera Cane. Pressing too vigorously can hurt the muscle, so start with treating the upper layers of skin first and then proceed to deeper fibers of the targeted muscle.

The Thera Cane is a very handy tool that can be used to treat the myofascial pains in those areas which are hard to reach by the hands (middle back and posterior thighs, etc.).

5. Management With Balls

Mindful breathing as described under "Management through Foam Rollers" can also be used when you are using balls. One of the most comfortable and handy ways to release muscle knots is by using balls on these painful points. You can choose between a wide range of balls to self-release your painful muscles. It can be a tennis ball, a massage (therapeutic) ball, a wooden ball, a cork ball, a soft air ball or a peanut ball. You can use the balls on the floor e.g. for back, shoulders and neck or you can also use the ball on a table e.g. by rolling your arm over the ball.

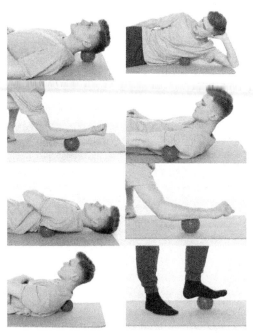

For shoulders and upper arms, you can also lean into the ball against a wall and roll your body up and down.

Tennis balls

A tennis ball is an easily available and handy option to self-treat myofascial pains. You can simply press these balls on the muscle knots and massage them just like the foam rollers, which we have covered in the previous chapter. Tennis balls can effectively treat muscle knots, which are present in deeper muscle layers. Pressing these knots with fingers or thumbs can lead to soreness in your fingers, and thus, a tennis ball is a great alternative.

The idea behind the tennis ball massage is to apply specific pressure on the painful knot in the muscle or over a tight fascia and feel the release. You can use a tennis ball to treat trigger points, tender points, or fascial distortion present on various parts of the body (neck, shoulder, back, arm, leg, etc.). By using a tennis ball, you can reach those painful areas which are not easily accessible with fingers and thumbs. To properly use a tennis ball over your painful area, place the tennis ball in a way that you can apply specific pressure on that area.

You can place a ball on the painful area or simply place the area over the tennis ball and press it. Whatever the position is, you should apply comfortable, controlled, but enough pressure over that painful myofascial area. It should elicit a "good pain" or also called "a release," which is satisfying in nature. Stay in an easy and relaxed position during the tennis ball release and feel the melting of a tight knot or distorted fascia beneath the ball. You can try the tennis ball massage several times a day, and each session can last for 2-5 minutes.

It is essential that you should not apply uncontrolled or unbearable pressure on tender myofascial areas, because it will cause no benefit to your muscles or fascia. You don't need to push your limits by hurting your muscles with excessive pressure. Just keep it simple, controlled, and pleasant.

A tennis ball is very beneficial to release myofascial pain in the neck, back, hips, calves, buttocks and thighs. You can also use it over your upper extremity and torso, but the pressure on these areas should be perfectly controlled.

Myofascial pain in the thighs can be managed by placing the ball between the thigh and the floor. Press the ball gently between your thigh and the floor to feel the release in the tight muscles.

Sometimes, it is hard to find the exact location of pain, and you should press the ball in the surrounding areas to explore the exact spot, to find the primary origin of pain. Sometimes, areas surrounding the painful muscle knots are also tight so, moving the tennis ball beneath these areas and massaging them will also alleviate the referral zones of myofascial pain.

Soft air balls
Air balls are called this simply because they have air inside them, so you can sink easily into the ball. If you have been to an inside children's play area, where the kids jump into a pool of soft balls: that's the type of ball I am talking about here.

The way you use these soft air balls is exactly the same as you would use a tennis ball.

Some people prefer softer balls. The soft balls come in all different sizes: from 4cm (1.5 inches) up to 25cm (10 inches).

Just experiment to see what your body and muscles like and what works best for you: tennis balls or soft balls.

These are also called therapeutic balls because of their extensive use in rehabilitations. These balls are available in various diameters, and the compressive strength of these balls also varies according to therapeutic usage. These balls are often present in black, red, blue, yellow, and green colors. Black colored massage balls have the highest compressive strengths, i.e. more pressure is required to compress them as compared to other colors, and green colored balls are the easiest to compress.

The techniques to use massage balls are very similar to tennis balls, but these balls provide more gentle pressure compared to the tennis balls. Because of their soft and compressible nature, these balls are safer to use on more tender and painful areas of the body.

Spiky balls
Some people prefer spiky balls, which also come in various sizes and colors, but these are not suitable for some areas of the body e.g. knees and neck. As a general rule, only people with strong muscles should use spiky balls. As a beginner, start with a soft air ball or tennis ball.

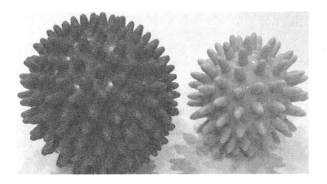

Wooden balls
These balls are made of wood and incompressible in nature. Myofascial pains, which are caused by trigger points in thighs, calves, and muscles of the back, are often hard to treat with compressible balls. Wooden balls provide more localized and more intense pressure to treat these myofascial pains, but the use of these balls is very limited because of the possible post-treatment soreness.

These balls are not compressible, and you should avoid using these balls if you have fibromyalgia. These balls are not suitable for delicate structures like pelvic organs and severely painful muscle knots.

Below is a picture of many different types of balls you can use, soft, wooden, tennis etc. You can buy these in a range of online stores.

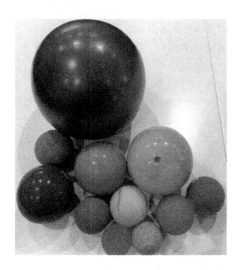

Peanut ball

The peanut ball is also called a double ball: 2 balls connected. These balls are especially good to use on neck, shoulders, back and feet but can be used anywhere on the body. You can use the balls whilst lying on a floor or leaning against a wall.

As shown on the picture below: you can simply put 2 balls e.g. tennis balls in a sock and tie a knot in the sock to keep the balls in place. This is especially handy if you do your upper back leaning against a wall as you can keep the end of the sock in your hand to keep the balls in place whilst you roll your body up and down the wall.

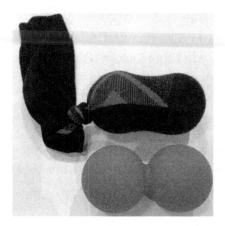

6. Management With Stretching

Simply stretching is a great way of releasing myofascial pain. Let us take a few minutes to look at different methods of stretching below:

Important: Always stretch slowly, as fascia doesn't like to be stretched quickly. Remember the cling film comparison: if you pull cling film apart too quickly, it will break. The same applies for your fascia: fascia can tear if stretched too quickly and so create extra pain. Always keep this in mind when doing any type of stretching.

Static stretching

This is the one you know, where you reach as far as you can and then try to push even further (bending over to touch your toes, for example).

Static stretching focuses on increasing the range of motion by pushing beyond it, whilst keeping the muscles fairly relaxed. It is beneficial for people who require a large range of motion, such as dancers. Static stretching can effectively treat myofascial pain arising from tight muscles.

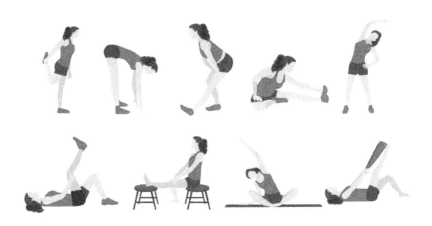

Passive or assisted stretching

This is very similar to static stretching, but either you or another person holds part of you in a stretched position. It feels great to have an assistant stretch you beyond your normal ranges of motion after a workout. However, pushing limits is not a smart idea, and it can cause an electromechanical delay (which means it takes longer from when the muscle starts to work to the time it actually produces a movement) after passive stretching.

Active stretching
You hold a position without any outside help, i.e. with your leg up in the air for around 10–15 seconds. While keeping the muscles on one side in contraction, you allow the muscles on the opposite side to relax and lengthen.

Resistance stretching
In this type of stretch, a muscle is contracted while you are stretching the muscle to its end ranges. That means the muscle will remain in a steady state of active contraction during the process of stretching. Remember, a muscle is stretched when both ends are moved far from each other. In the simple contraction of muscle, these two ends of muscles arc brought together, and the length of the muscle is shortened. In stretching, the length of the muscle is increased.

Resistance stretching is a combination of active muscle contraction and muscle stretching. For example, if you want to resistance stretch your bicep, you will contract your bicep, but rather than flexing the arm, you will extend it while keeping the bicep muscle in a contraction state. Similarly, if you want to resistance stretch your hamstring, you will contract the hamstring muscle, but you will not flex the knee. You will extend the knee while maintaining the contraction in hamstring muscles.

Resistance stretching helps in increasing the strength of muscles while increasing their flexibility. So, it targets the most important characteristics of a muscle by keeping the balance between muscle fibers. Research has shown that resistance stretching leads to more activation of muscle fibers, as well as more flexibility in targeted muscles.

You can use resistance stretches to treat myofascial pains, but it requires great control of muscles and a deep understanding of resistance stretches. It is suggested that the resistance stretch should be performed under the guidance of an expert physiotherapist or an osteopath until you are trained, because uncontrolled movements can further hurt the already painful muscle.

PNF stretching

Short for Proprioceptive Neuromuscular Facilitation, PNF was initially developed as a method for rehabilitating stroke victims. You go to the end of the range of motion and then contract your muscle (by pushing against someone holding you in a fixed position) for around 5 seconds only, before relaxing and possibly going further in the stretch before repeating.

Isometric stretching

An isometric contraction is one without movement; this will give you a clue as to what this type of stretching consists of. You go to the end of the range of motion, contract your muscles for around 7–15 seconds, relax and repeat.

A common example is the calf stretch at the wall, where you are pushing against the wall and not going anywhere.

Ballistic stretching

This is almost as dynamic as it sounds, using explosive movements to push the body into a stretched position and allowing the elastic recoil of the body to pull it back again.

It consists of lots of bouncing, falling into lunges, swinging the arms rapidly, and other fast movements.

Dynamic stretching

This also involves movement, but in a much slower and controlled manner. You never go past your natural range of movement, and it seems to be more geared toward increasing mobility rather than specifically increasing the range of motion.

The movements include a variety of swinging limbs, twists, and natural movements.

Active isolated

In this system of stretching, you move into a stretch by contracting the muscles on the other side of the body (i.e. the quads, when stretching the hamstrings) and hold it for a very short amount of time. The theory is that you avoid triggering the stretch reflex by only holding it for 2 seconds.

Loaded stretching

When performing loaded stretching, you take your muscle through its whole range whilst it simultaneously contracts. The reason that it is contracting is that there is a weight pulling it, and your limb is resisting that. Your limb and the weight are both going in the same direction, which moves you into a stretch, but your muscles have the brakes on, which means they are continuously contracted.

General Warm-Up Stretches

These stretches are amazing for waking up in the morning, warming up for stretching or exercise, or just to wind down from a busy day. They get the body moving as a whole, increasing blood and lymph circulation, warming the muscles up, and also get you in the mood for stretching.

Aim to be gentle and relaxed while keeping the body engaged. Do not tense your muscles 100%, but ease into the movements; the focus is to warm up rather than to stretch strongly. You can increase the amount of tension in your muscles as you get more warmed up.

I recommend that you do them roughly in the order given, as the more general, whole-body stretches are at the beginning, and then the ones toward the end are targeted to more specific areas. Because they do involve a larger area than some of the more specific stretches that we cover later on, it is important to create tension in a lot of muscles at once.

Note: If you start your myofascial release session with a few warm-up stretches, it can be a great idea to do a couple of the same warm-up stretches again at the end of your session. Why? Because there are a few things that reflect your changes back to you as well as a specific movement such as a stretch. See if it is easier to do these stretches at the end of your stretching session, and also notice whether your posture has changed and how you feel different. You may notice a difference in the range of motion, ease of movement, fluidity, balance, or coordination, for example.

Further Stretches for Myofascial pain

These stretches are perfect for people wanting to generally improve their posture, as they focuse on the tight areas that frequently pull people out of their naturally healthy alignment.

CHILD'S POSE WITH RESISTANCE
Main area and muscles stretched
Stretches the upper back and upper arms.
Technique
Get onto your hands and knees and keeping a slight bend in your elbows, pull back your hands down into the ground, with your palms flat. As you continuously pull your hands down into the ground and back toward you, smoothly sit back on your heels. Your knees are on the floor, and your stomach is close to your knees. Your arms are outstretched, and palms are down.
Technique tips
If it is in your comfortable range, then bring the hands further forward and if it is too difficult, move your hands a little closer to your knees.

HIP FLEXOR LOW LUNGE
Main area and muscles stretched
Stretches the hip flexors.
Technique
Crouch as if you were getting into the starting position for a race, with both hands on the floor, and then try to open your legs as far as you can to put them far away from your hands. Keep your buttocks high in the air as you lower your hips down and lift your head as far as you can comfortably go.
Technique tips
To generate even more resistance, you can pull your back leg down into the ground from the very beginning of the stretch. You are stretching the front of the hip of the leg that is behind you.
Suggested number of reps in one set
7–10 on each side.

SATELLITE ARMS
Main area and muscles stretched
Stretches the chest and the upper back.
Technique

In this stretch, the arms rotate around you, with your palms always facing the body. Start with your arms straight down and in front of the body. Tensing your chest and shoulders, move your arms out to the sides and around behind you to stretch your chest.

Then tensing your back, move your arms back around to the front again, stretching your upper back. Keep your hands close to your body. Moving your arms backward and then forward counts as one rep.

Technique tips

This stretch is unusual in that you stretch in both directions, so it is really two stretches rolled into one. Because of this, you have to remember to keep the resistance in the correct area in order for the stretch to work. Try not to raise your shoulders.

Suggested number of reps in one set

7–10.

SITTING GLUTE STRETCH WITH STRAP

Main area and muscles stretched

Stretches the glutes.

Technique

Sit in a chair and make a loop with a yoga strap, belt, or towel. Have one leg in the air, bent at 90°, with the hand of the same side holding the thigh under the knee to stabilize it. Place the loop around the foot and swing your foot outward as far as it can comfortably go. As you continue to pull your foot outward, smoothly pull your foot, with the yoga strap, across your body towards the opposite shoulder.

Technique tips

Please note that this stretch is all about pivoting, rather than the whole leg moving out to the side. Therefore, the thigh and knee stay in roughly the same place, while only the foot and upper leg move.

Suggested number of reps in one set

7–10 on each side.

CHEST PULL BACK

Main area and muscles stretched

Stretches the chest and the front of your shoulders.

Technique

Clasp your hands behind your back (or you can hold a yoga strap) with straight arms and hunch your shoulders forward. Tense your chest continuously as you lift your hands and open your chest.

Technique tips

To increase the area that is stretched, you can also tense the front of your neck and your upper chest and look upward at the same time as pulling your arms back.

Suggested number of reps in one set

7–10.

HIP FLEXOR PUSH-UP

Main area and muscles stretched

Stretches the hip flexors.

Technique

Get into a full push-up position and push your hips high up into the air. Tensing the front of your hips and abdomen, lower your hips toward the ground against that continuous tension, simultaneously looking up. Return easily to the starting position and repeat.

Technique tips

If this is too hard, then you can do it in a kneeling push-up position, in which case you should let your feet point up into the air.

Please note that although it looks a bit like the yoga Cobra pose, it has a different effect, as the stretch happens while you are moving, and you keep the resistance on in the front of your thighs in order to ensure your hip flexors are being stretched. In addition, do not let your thighs touch the ground and make sure you do not hold the pose but keep moving through it.

Suggested number of reps in one set

5–7.

SITTING ABDUCTOR SQUEEZE

Main area and muscles stretched

Stretches the abductors.

Technique

Sit with your knees bent in front of your chest, feet together, arms around your legs, and hands clasped (fingers interlinked). Start with your knees as far apart as they can go, and then as your knees push out continuously, straighten your arms and squeeze inward to stretch your abductors.

Technique tips

Try not to raise your shoulders as you do this, particularly if you have shoulder and neck tension.

Suggested number of reps in one set
7–10.

CAT STRETCH
Main area and muscles stretched
Stretches the whole back.
Technique
Get onto your hands and knees and tense your back as you bend it down, lowering your belly button toward the floor. Keep the tension on as you arch your back up as far as you can go. From there, you can push your back all the way down again and move fluidly from one to the other. Lowering and raising your back once counts as one rep.
Technique tips
Do not push through any pain, and also remember to look up when your back is down and down when your back is up.
Suggested number of reps in one set
7-10.

LATS ON THE FLOOR
Main area and muscles stretched
Stretches the back and the lats (muscle which is present on both sides of our back) especially.
Technique
It starts by stabilizing your body on all fours and by keeping your elbows on the floor, underneath your shoulders, and roll your arms onto their sides. Keep the palms towards each other and your forearms parallel. Pull your hands down and back toward you into the floor, and smoothly sit back onto your heels.
Technique tips
Try to keep your back flat like a table and let your shoulders stay away from your ears as much as possible. To intensify the stretch, move your hands further forward and to lessen the intensity, move them closer to your knees.
Suggested number of reps in one set
7–10.

Active Isolated Stretch (AIS)

Muscles cannot extend without fascia. There is a three-dimensional fibrous matrix that provides interconnections throughout all cells of the body.

Fascial distortion by trauma, aging, posture, hormonal changes, or metabolic disturbances disrupts the body homeostasis.

Left untreated, these conditions promote detrimental contractures, inflammation, lymphatic congestion, peripheral vascular obstruction, hypertension, and a host of other disease states.

AIS is widely used as a therapeutic myofascial technique termed the Mattes Method.

This method promotes functional and physiologic restoration of muscles, tendons, vertebrae, ligaments, and joints, facilitating healthier superficial and deep fascial planes.

The Mattes Method enables optimal myofascial stretching of isolated muscles without activating a protective reflex contraction.

The Mattes Method uses a gradual stretch of maximum 2 seconds, promoting a full range of flexibility and motion without activating muscle group contraction.

Example of wrist flexors

Wrist flexors are the muscles that bring the wrist towards the forearm.

1. To stretch the wrist extensors, the arm and elbow are held in extension, and the first move is a voluntary flexion of the wrist, which contracts the wrist flexors, thereby relaxing the wrist extensors.
2. The initial voluntary contraction creates a gentle stretch with less than 1 pound of pressure toward the endpoint of the range.
3. This is followed by no greater than a 2-second stretch of the flexed wrist.
4. Continue repeating this same isolated muscle stretch up to 10 times, with each subsequent stretch to achieve an incremental

gain of a few degrees of motion without eliciting a contraction of opposing muscle.

5. Always return the area being stretched to the starting position before continuing the prescribed repetitions.

6. This results in better hemodynamics (blood circulation), more lymphatic drainage, and waste removal, as well as empowering the neural response.

7. Monitor the stretch reflex carefully as the tissue is stretched to the point of "light irritation," then release the tension to prevent reversal contraction of the muscles/fascia being stretched.

7. Management With Massage

Self-massage based on Chinese and Thai techniques
In China, self-massage is also called health-care message (bao Jian tui na), while in ancient times, it was known as dao yin an mo (abducting and leading massage). Such self-massage therapy has a long history in China, going back literally thousands of years. One can see examples of such dao yin mo exercises and manipulations drawn on the Ma Wang Tui scrolls dating from the Western Han dynasty (206 BC-24 AD). The ancient Chinese combined massage manipulations, breathing exercises and mental relaxation, concentration, and visualization to maximize and restore health to the human body.

Chinese mythology considers wellness as a state of balance, and self-massage is one simple and free way of maintaining and restoring that balance. It is a basic belief of Chinese medicine that the internal organs of the body are connected to every part of the body by a network of large and small channels. The larger of these channels are called channels and vessels, while the smaller channels are called network vessels. These channels and network vessels are the highways and byways for the circulation and movement of the body's energy, called qi, and blood. This energy or qi and blood is created in the internal organs and then sent out to the rest of the body to nourish and empower it.

Rolfing
Rolfing is a massage technique proposed by Dr. Ida Rolf. Her famous quote about rolfing is "it doesn't matter how deep you go, the only

thing matters is how you go deep." In rolfing massage, you will start pressing and kneading the superficial layers of skin while feeling the release in a painful area. As you feel that there is enough release in the upper layers, you will press with increased pressure to target the deeper layers of skin until you reach the painful muscle. You will treat the muscle in the same way. Rolfing is an advanced massage skill that requires proper certification, but the basic concept is easy to follow, i.e. treat the outermost layers first and feel the release.

Self-massage methods to treat myofascial pain of the neck, upper back, and upper extremity

1. Finger pressing tender points on the back: First, search by touch for tender points on the sides of the spine on the back. Then finger press and knead these tender points with the knuckles of both thumbs 100-200 times.
2. Pressing & kneading: With the tips of both thumbs, search for tender points on the outsides of and just below the knees. Then press and knead these with strong force 100-200 times.
3. Pressing & kneading: With the tips of both thumbs, press and knead the points on the backs of the feet 100-200 times.
4. Circular rubbing the upper & middle abdomen: With one palm, circularly rub around the midpoint of the upper abdomen and the navel clockwise for 3-5 minutes each.
5. Obliquely rubbing the lateral coastal regions: With both palms, rub both lateral coastal regions from the armpits to the sides of the abdomen to and fro to produce a sensation of heat.
6. Pressing & kneading painful points on knees: With the tips of both thumbs, press and knead the points on the lateral sides of both knees in front of and below the small head of the fibula (outer side of the knee) approximately 100 times each.
7. Pressing & kneading: With the tips of both thumbs, press and knead Zu San Li (located three inches below the lower outside edge of the kneecap) approximately 100 times each.
8. Press & knead the back of the head: Place the pads or the tips of both thumbs securely on the points on the back of the head. This point is located one body inch (i.e. approximately the width of the thumb knuckle) above the hairline in the dip between the skull and the long muscles at the back of the neck. Press these forcefully more than ten times, followed by circular kneading.

For the best effect, one should create a sensation of mild soreness and distention in the local area.

9. Washing the face with the hands: Rub the palms of the hands briskly against each other until they are warm. Then place the palms tightly against the forehead, rubbing forcefully down to the lower jaws and along the edges of the lower jaw. Then continue rubbing on upwards past the fronts of the ears and the temples to the midpoint of the forehead. Repeat this procedure 20-30 times until a warm sensation is felt all over the face.

10. Kneading & circular rubbing the neck and nape: With one palm, knead and circularly rub the affected side of the neck and nape of the neck from the base of the skull to the upper back. Then turn the head towards the shoulder on the affected side until there is a feeling of heat, comfort is attained in the local area, and the pain is relieved.

11. Grasping the nape: With the thumb, index, and middle fingers of one hand, grasp the muscles of the nape of the neck on the affected side from the base of the skull to the shoulder several times.

12. Rubbing the nape: With one palm, rub the nape of the neck on the affected side from the base of the skull to the upper back and shoulder until there is a feeling of heat.

13. Pressing & kneading the junction of head and neck: With the tips of both thumbs, press and knead the points just slightly above the posterior hairline and in the depression between the mastoid process (area of skull just behind the jaw) and the long muscles at the back of the neck 30-50 times. Rotate the head while kneading.

14. Pressing & kneading Tian Zong (SI 11): With the tip of the middle finger, press and knead the point in the center of the scapula below its spine 100-200 times to produce a feeling of soreness and distention in the upper back. At the same time, rotate the head slowly, starting out with small circles and expanding to larger circles. A relaxed feeling should be felt in the neck.

15. Pressing & kneading the tender points: With the tip of one thumb, press and knead any tender points on the neck, beginning with weak pressure and gradually increasing to strong. Then pluck the point for approximately 2-3 minutes

16. Pushing the heavenly pillar bones: With the index and middle fingers of one hand, push the line on the nape of the neck from

the midpoint of the hairline to the bulging bone (C7) at the base of the neck 30-50 times.

17. Pressing & kneading tender points: With the tip of the thumb or the tips of the index and middle fingers, press and knead any tender point on the neck until the pain is relieved.

18. Grasping & rubbing the arm: With the thumb, index, and middle fingers of the other hand, grasp the outer and inner sides of the affected arm from the shoulder to the wrist several times. Then, with the palm, rub both sides of the arm to produce a feeling of heat.

19. Kneading the shoulder: With the heel of the palm of the other hand, knead every side of the affected shoulder, beginning with weak pressure and gradually applying stronger pressure for 3-5 minutes.

20. Pinching & grasping the muscles of the shoulder: With the thumb, index, and middle fingers of the other hand, pinch and grasp the muscles of the affected shoulder for 3-5 minutes, grasping more on the deltoid muscle on the lateral side of the shoulder. The deltoid muscle is present above the bicep muscle.

21. Pinching & grasping the upper arm: With the thumb, index, and middle fingers of the other hand, pinch and grasp the muscles of the anterior and posterior sides of the affected upper arm from the shoulder to the elbow 30-50 times.

22. Pressing & kneading tender points: With the tip of the thumb or middle finger, press and knead any tender points around the shoulder, beginning with weak pressure and gradually pressing more strongly. At the same time, mobilize the shoulder for 2-3 minutes.

23. Pressing & kneading the lateral side of the elbow and forearm: With the thumb, press and knead the lateral side of the elbow, forearm, and wrist of the affected arm. Repeat this procedure 5-10 times.

24. Pressing & kneading tender points: With the thumb, press and knead any tender points on the lateral side of the affected elbow for 2-3 minutes.

25. Pressing & kneading the forearm: With the palm of the other hand, press and knead the affected forearm on the palmar side from the wrist to the elbow 5-10 times.

26. Pressing & kneading the area of the carpal tunnel: With the tip of the thumb, press and knead the affected wrist and surface of the

palm, beginning with weak force and ending with strong, for 2-3 minutes.

27. Rotation & traction of the wrist: With the opposite hand, hold the fingers of the affected hand. Then extend the wrist backward and flex it forward as far as possible approximately ten times in each direction. Next, rotate the wrist approximately ten times in each direction and finally pull the wrist straight forward, tractioning it 3-5 times.

28. Rubbing the palm & forearm: With the other palm, rub the affected forearm from the surface of the palm to the elbow to and fro 10-20 times.

Self-massage techniques for low back and lower limbs

Due to humankind's assumption of an upright posture, more mechanical pressure is applied to the lower back region than most other parts of the body. Therefore, a lumbar sprain is a very common complaint in daily life. The main causes of a lumbar sprain are carrying heavy objects, trying to lift too heavy objects with the back instead of the legs, sudden twisting of the waist, and injury due to fall or strike directly on or to the low back. For best results, Chinese self-massage should be used as soon after the acute injury as possible. The longer we ignore the process, the more likely that acute lumbar sprain may become chronic low back pain, which then is enduring and difficult to treat.

Chinese self-massage is a very effective method for treating a lumbar sprain. Generally, two to three treatments with Chinese self-massage can cure acute lumbar sprain.

Usually, patients with this complaint experience at least some symptoms immediately after the sprain, such as severe lumbar pain, limitation of and difficulty moving when sitting, lying, turning over and sitting up from bed, and worsening of the pain when coughing, sneezing, or taking a deep breath. If the case is mild, there may be no obvious lumbar pain immediately after the sprain, but they may experience progressive pain or limited lumbar movement several hours or 1-2 days later.

Lumbar pain

1. Pressing & kneading the lumbar region: With the heel of one palm, press and knead the lumbar muscles on the affected side, moving from top to bottom as one presses and kneads. Do this for 2-5 minutes to help the lumbar muscles to relax.

2. Pressing & kneading tender points: With the tip of one thumb, press and knead any tender points and the area around such tender points in the lumbar region. The force should go from weak to strong but bearable. Continue pressing and kneading for 2-3 minutes. It is a good sign if this tenderness is relieved after pressing and kneading these tender points.

3. Rubbing the lumbar region: With the side of one palm, rub the lumbar muscles on the affected side up and down to produce a sensation of heat. Then, with the center of the palm, rub the lumbosacral region transversely to and fro to produce a sensation of heat. Some massage ointment, such as Tiger Balm or Temple of Heaven, should be applied to the area prior to rubbing to improve the curative effect.

Chronic lumbar muscle strain mainly refers to a chronic injury of the soft tissues of the low back, such as the muscles, ligaments, and connecting tissue in the lumbosacral region. Chronic low back strain is the main cause of chronic lumbago. Chronic lumbar muscle strain is mainly due to long-term muscle fatigue and repetitive micro trauma, such as from working in an asymmetric or ergonomically inappropriate posture.

A chronic lumbar muscle strain may also be caused by an acute lumbar sprain, which has not been treated soon enough or completely, or which has reoccurred many times. Thus, acute lumbar sprain may evolve into chronic lumbar muscle strain. In most cases of chronic lumbar muscle strain, there is mild soreness or a vague, lingering pain at ordinary times.

This pain then becomes more severe when the person either becomes fatigued or the weather becomes overcast and rainy. This pain may be located on one or both sides or in the middle of the lumbosacral area. The tender area is comparatively large, and there are no fixed tender spots. In addition, there is usually no disturbance or limitation in the movement of the waist and low back area.

Treating chronic lumbar muscle strain with Chinese self-massage is less effective than treating an acute lumbar sprain. Sometimes, Chinese self-massage does get marked results after several treatments, but unfortunately, this condition may also easily relapse when the person gets fatigued or during cold, damp weather. Thus, in order to be effective, one must persevere in regularly performing Chinese self-massage for the treatment of chronic lumbar muscle strain. Otherwise, good effects cannot be obtained.

Lumbar muscles
1. Pressing & kneading the lumbar region: With the heel of each palm, press and knead the lumbosacral muscles on both sides of the low back, moving from top to bottom at the same time as pressing & kneading. Do this for 3-5 minutes to produce a feeling of soreness and distention. The force of pressing and kneading should be deep and strong.
2. Plucking the lumbar muscles: With the tips of both thumbs, press and knead the lumbosacral muscles on both sides of the spine and then pluck the muscles like plucking the string of a guitar, moving from top to bottom at the same time as plucking. Do this for 3-5 minutes.
3. Grasping the lumbar muscles: With the five fingers of each hand, grasp the lumbar muscles on both sides of the spine from top to bottom 5-10 times.
4. Rubbing the lumbosacral region: With both palms, rub the lumbosacral muscles on both sides of the spine up and down to produce a feeling of heat. Then, with one palm, transversely rub the lumbosacral region to and fro to also produce a feeling of heat. One should apply some massage ointment to the area before rubbing.

Knees
The joints of the knees are among the largest and most complex joints in the body. Because they bear such a heavy burden and are subjected to such a wide variety of forces coming from all different angles, injury of the knee joint is very common. These knee joint injuries lead to acute and chronic myofascial pains around the joint and associated areas. There are several kinds of knee joint injury, depending on which tissues within or around the knee have been injured. The most common ones are injury of the collateral ligament,

inflammation of the joint capsule due to trauma, and injury of the meniscus of the knee joint.

It is important to note that the back of the knee is a delicate area of your body packed with sensitive nerves and fascia, especially the back of the knee. Always be careful with massaging your knee and never press too hard.

The main symptoms of acute knee joint injury are pain and swelling in the knee joint and restriction of the movement of the knee. In the early stage of injury, Chinese self-massage manipulations should be applied with weak and gentle force to disperse swelling and relieve pain. As the pain and swelling are alleviated, the self-massage can become gradually stronger, and small range movement of the knee joint can be gradually added.

1. Pressing & kneading tender points: With the tip of the thumb, press and knead any tender points found near the knee joint for 3-5 minutes.
2. Pushing & kneading the knee region: With the heel of one palm, knead the area of the knee, moving while kneading from the thigh to lower leg along with the anterior, medial, and lateral sides of the knee 3-5 times on each side.
3. Grasping the lower limb: With the five fingers of one hand, grasp the anterior, posterior, medial, and lateral sides of the affected lower limb from the thigh to the foot 3-5 times on each side.
4. Kneading & circular rubbing of the injured area: With one palm, gently knead or circularly rub the injured area until a feeling of heat is felt.
5. Twisting & kneading the knee joint: Place one palm on each side of the affected knee joint, twisting and kneading the knee joint with both palms like twisting a rope. While twisting, move along both sides of the knee from the thigh to the lower leg approximately ten times. This twisting should be quick, while the moving should be slow.

Ankles
The ankle joint is the easiest joint in the body to sprain. These sprains often lead to myofascial pains and trigger points around the ankle joint. Most sprained ankles occur when walking on an uneven road,

downstairs or on a downhill path, running, or jumping. Eversion or turning outward of the ankle is common. Self-massage is effective for treating a sprain or partial rupture of the ankle. However, Chinese self-massage is contraindicated if there is a complete rupture of the ligament, fracture of the ankle bones, or dislocation of the ankle joint. Therefore, if the ankle is severely injured with severe swelling and pain, one should see a professional health care practitioner.

1. Pushing & kneading the lateral or medial side of the lower leg: With the heel of the palm, knead the outer or inner side of the lower leg, moving at the time of kneading from the knee to the ankle 3-5 times on each side of the leg.
2. Grasping the lower leg: With the five fingers of one hand, grasp the lateral or medial side of the lower leg from the knee to the ankle 3-5 times on each side of the leg.
3. Circular rubbing the injured area: With the center of the palm, circularly rub the injured area where it is painful for 3-5 minutes.
4. Rubbing the injured area: With the center of the palm, rub the injured area up and down to produce a feeling of heat. The force of rubbing toward the center of the body should be strong, while the force toward the toes of the foot should be weak so as to subdue swelling.
5. Rotating the ankle joint: Hold the tip of the foot in one hand and cup the heel of the foot with the other. Then rotate the ankle clockwise and counterclockwise 10-20 times in each direction.
6. Tractioning the ankle joint: Hold the foot with both hands in the same way as rotating the ankle joint described above, pulling and extending the ankle joint after rotating it, fully extending the ankle joint 3-5 times.

Some Other Common Massage Techniques
Massage is most people's favorite because it can reduce the anxiety that contributes to reducing muscle tension. Massage can also increase blood flow to an area, which may hasten to heal. Performing simple self-myofascial release moves daily with the foam roller can keep muscles fluid, prevent future issues, and offer many other benefits.

I have tried to address the self-massage in detail. The heading is Chinese and Thai massage, but if you want to follow modern or more therapeutic massages, I am going to throw light on it too. Below are some important therapeutic or western massage techniques. These techniques are the same as I described earlier, but the difference lies between the terminologies. You can apply the exact self-massage on the above-mentioned areas by slightly manipulating the direction of the force.

Cross friction and deep friction massage
Cross friction massage is moving or manipulating the skin and tissue beneath it through the help of an external force that is applied perpendicular to the direction of tissue. Deep friction massage is stimulating and manipulating the deeper fibers of muscles regardless of the direction of applied force. You can perform self-massage in the cross friction or deep friction way to manage myofascial pains, which come from deep sources such as paraspinal muscles etc.

Transverse friction massage
Transverse friction massage is the application of force along the direction of tissues to be treated to help in managing the tightness and myofascial pain.

Skin rolling and skin tapping
These are also some other types of massage technique which help in improving the tissue turgor and extensibility. Remember, I told you in previous chapters that adhesions and immobilization of tissue can lead to myofascial pain syndrome? Well, these two techniques are very effective in managing these issues.

8. Management With Reflexology Techniques

The origins
Reflexology is the process of applying pressure to the hands or feet, which correspond to certain parts of the body. Although it is commonly believed that reflexology came from China, there is evidence that it was also used in Ancient Egyptian, Babylonian, and Native North American cultures. A carving at a physician's tomb in Saqqara in Egypt (dating to 2350 BC) depicts what looks like both a foot and hand reflexology treatment.

Foot Reflexology Chart

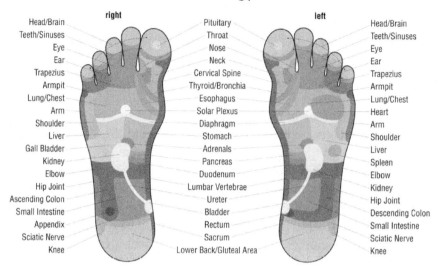

The longitudinal zones

The reflexology used in the West today has its origin in nineteenth-century Russian and German scientific inquiry. An American, Dr. William Fitzgerald, who studied reflex theory while working in Vienna, consolidated some of this research along with his own theories and published the book *Zone Therapy* in 1917.

Fitzgerald divided the body into ten equal longitudinal zones of energy, running from the feet, up the legs, down the arms, and up into the brain. The zones were numbered from one to five, from the middle of the body to the outside, on both sides. Fitzgerald theorized that any impairment to the free flow of life-force energy or chi would affect the vital parts of the body and the organs within that specific zone.

Reflex zones of the foot

Fitzgerald taught zone therapy to a friend and colleague, Dr. Shelby Riley. However, it was Riley's associate, Eunice Ingham, a physical therapist, who became particularly enthusiastic about the work. Ingham experimented with the effects of working on different areas of the feet in relation to the ten longitudinal zones until she was able to map the entire body on the feet.

Practicing reflexology techniques

Because the reflex areas are minute, they must be stimulated directly and precisely. Circular friction-massage or back-and-forth rubbing is not as effective as pinching an area, rotating on a point, or thumb-walking.

Pinching

Pinching is exactly what it sounds like – you pinch with your index finger and thumb to precisely stimulate an area. The thumb is usually the tool that stimulates the reflex zone, while the index finger stabilizes the thumb on the other side of the hand or foot.

Rotating on a point

For this technique, place your thumb on the reflex zone and your other fingers around the back of the foot or hand. Press into the area with your thumb, supporting the pressure with your fingers from the other side. Then rotate your thumb as you continue to hold the pressure.

This technique may take a little more practice. It is often described as using the thumb to crawl like a caterpillar over the reflex zone. Place the pad of your thumb on your opposite palm. Now bend the knuckle so that you roll up to the tip of your thumb.

Next, flatten your thumb again, but move it forward about 0.5 cm (¼ inch). Never let your thumb lose contact with the skin. Repeat the action over your palm several times until it becomes an easy, repetitive action.

9. Management With Heat

Heat or thermotherapy is the use of heat for the therapeutic purpose. Heating a sore area is a very ancient technique because it helps to increase the blood supply in that area, and thus, painful mediators are removed very efficiently. Heating can be done by electrical hot packs, or it can simply be done by using household hot water bottles, warm baths, electric heating pads, electric blankets or even through massage. Whatever the principle is, heating should be done in a controlled and cautious way because overheating can cause burns and blistering. Thermotherapy is a proven method to treat myofascial pains and trigger points.

For some people heat and ice is used alternately, each for 10 to 15 minutes works well too.

10.Management With Cryotherapy

Cryotherapy or icing (cold therapy) is using cold for therapeutic purposes. Cold therapy is used in the first 1-3 days of an injury or soreness to prevent inflammation and pain. Cryotherapy in myofascial pain syndrome has shown miraculous results, and researchers are focusing on using cryotherapy as a standard to treat myofascial pain syndrome. Stationary application of cold for more than 2 minutes provides the effects of heat, so it should be avoided in recent injuries. Generally, use cold therapy for 10 to 15 minutes, any longer and it won't give you any extra benefits.

11.Management With Electrotherapy

Electrotherapy is the use of physiological currents to treat myofascial pains and other illnesses. There are a variety of user-friendly devices that can help you in self-treatment of trigger points, tender points, muscle tightness, muscle spasm, and all those conditions which lead to myofascial pain syndrome.

TENS

The first and most effective device of this list is TENS. Transcutaneous Electrical Nervous Stimulation (TENS) is based on low-frequency currents, which help in managing pain related to nerves, muscles, and fascia. Pain is actually the perception that is carried to our brain from the source. The pain is perceived by nociceptors, which are the receptors of pain in our skin. A TENS device consists of a user-friendly machine and four skin pads, which can be attached at the site of pain. 5-15 minutes of application of TENS 2-3 times a day can reduce myofascial pain considerably.

Interferential current

This device is very similar to TENS, but it is based on medium frequency currents. The use of the interferential device is proven in the case of myofascial pain and other neuromuscular injuries. It has a user-friendly device along with four attachable skin pads similar to TENS. 5-15 minutes application of IF current 2-3 times a day can reduce myofascial pain considerably.

Electrical hot packs

I have dedicated a complete section to discussing the benefits and uses of heat to treat myofascial pains. Electrical hot packs are very handy units to provide thermotherapy at home or in clinical settings. You can simply buy an affordable electrical hot pack and apply it to the sore and painful area for 10-15 mins 2-3 times a day.

Electrical cold packs and sprays

Similar to electrical hot packs, there are various cryotherapy sprays and electrical cold packs to manage myofascial pains and other neuromusculoskeletal injuries at home. You can simply buy an affordable electrical cold pack and apply it to the sore and painful area for 10-15 mins 2-3 times a day.

12. The Nutritional Aspects of Treating Myofascial Pain at Home

A balanced diet helps in effectively preventing myofascial pains by properly supplying the muscles with essential nutrients. It is evident that people with eating disorders suffer more from myofascial pains because their muscles are easily fatigued, and healing is very slow in these people. Moreover, junk food and over-eating causes fat accumulation in muscles, which hinders the proper functioning of muscles in our bodies,

A balanced diet incorporates all the essential nutritional components that are important in the proper functioning of our body systems. These nutritional components are divided into micro- and macro-nutrients.

The first thing you can do to prevent or treat myofascial pains is a lifestyle change, which requires a good diet and plenty of muscle training. Researchers have shown that a balanced diet prevents the accumulation of toxins, which can trigger the myofascial pains in our bodies.

A detailed discussion on macro and micronutrients

If you want to prevent or treat myofascial pain in the most effective way, you should know all the necessary components from which our diet is made. Your diet leads to your health, and many people experience myofascial pains because they have irregular dietary habits or they eat too much junk food, which leads to inflammation and toxicity of the myofascial structure. You have to eat a balanced diet and to balance your diet; you must know the basic building blocks of a healthy diet. There are two broad categories of nutrients, which are called the macro and micronutrients. Let's discuss these nutrients in detail:

Macro-Nutrients
As the name implies, macronutrients are the essential nutrients that comprise a more significant portion of our daily diet. These are essential because they form the foundation of daily caloric intake, and these are rich in energy. Macronutrients are three in types:
- Protein
- Fats
- Carbohydrates

Protein
Protein is the most critical type of macronutrient. The most important sources of protein are whey protein isolates, casein protein, salmon, tuna, chicken, turkey, beef, mutton, dairy, egg white, and some fruits/vegetables as well. A diet which comprises of high levels of protein can provide more advantages in getting lean muscle mass over those diets which lack sufficient amounts of protein. Protein is also an essential precursor of our enzymes, and our blood also has some essential types of proteins. So, having a high protein regime is a good idea to get a ripped physique as well as low body fat.

Fats
Fats are also called lipids and are essential energy supplies for the human body. Fats contain nine calories per gram, which are more than double the protein and carbohydrates (4 calories per gram). This is the reason that the body naturally stores fats as an emergency supply when we undergo calorie deficit dieting. The most significant benefit of storing fat as an emergency supply is it's hard to break and easy to consume characteristic.

There are different classifications of fats. Mono and polyunsaturated fatty acids are the highest quality fatty acids that are present in olive oils, some other plant oils, and some fish oils. Saturated fats are also essential to consume because of our hormones; mostly, the sex hormones are based on saturated fatty acids, which can be found in some animal and plant products. The worst type of fatty acids are trans-fatty acids, which to be avoided because of very harmful effects on our bodies.

A well-balanced diet should have fats in 0.5 grams per pound of bodyweight proportion, and zero consumption of any fat as achieved in some inferior yet trendy fat loss diets should be avoided because of severe health risks.

Carbohydrates
Carbohydrates are also termed as sugars, and the most consumed type of macronutrients around the globe are actually carbs. Carbohydrates can be low, medium, and high glycemic. Some carbs are simple, yet others are complex. A diet must have low and medium glycemic carbs such as oatmeal, honey, and fruits, but carbs having high glycemic indexes such as processed sugars and soda should be avoided. High glycemic carbs cause a rapid spike in blood sugar levels, and thus, it can lead to diabetes. However, complex high glycemic carbs can be utilized post-workout because they are essential to replenish the burnt glycogen storage in a human body after exercise.

Carbohydrates are those macronutrients that can be cycled, and the calorie deficit cyclic diet should periodize the carbohydrate intake to get maximum results with minimum leptin production and long-lasting results. Luckily, a balanced diet is well designed to provide all the essential carbs, yet cycling them in this diet provides rapid and long-lasting fat loss in a short duration of time.

Micro-nutrients
This category of nutrients in our daily diet comprises of those salts, minerals, and vitamins which are present in food inherently, or we can take them as a supplement. Iron, magnesium, calcium, potassium, and vitamins are some examples. Some of them are required in trace amounts, yet they are essential for the proper regulation of the body's essential cycles.

Vitamins are available in fruits and green leafy vegetables. Eating plenty of raw fruits and vegetables can effectively target the daily requirements of many essential vitamins, which can help in the proper functioning of our muscles. Vitamin B12 is very important in the proper healing of our muscles, and it is present in green leafy vegetables (broccoli, Spinach, etc.) and also in carrots. Apple is also a great source of Vitamin B12. This vitamin is a special mention because lots of clinical research concluded that Vitamin B12 helps in preventing myofascial pain syndromes. Similarly, Vitamin C, Vitamin K, and other essential vitamins play important roles in optimized muscular performance. There are many vitamin brands available, but the best source of getting these vitamins is raw dietary food (vegetables and fruits).

Iron and potassium are the two most important minerals which are essential for the proper contraction of muscles. Iron is present in green leafy vegetables (especially in spinach), and banana is a great source of potassium.

Muscle cramps and trigger points are often caused by depleted calcium and vitamin D levels. Calcium is present in dairy products and eggs. Vitamin D can be taken as a dietary supplement, but sunlight is also a great source of Vitamin D.

Importance of proper water intake
Our muscle is made up of protein, and when a muscle contracts, complex interactions occur between muscle fibers and filaments. These interactions are controlled by various minerals (calcium and potassium, and sodium), and proper homeostasis is essential to keep up the balance between these interactions. Homeostasis is the steady-state of the body in which every unit of our body acts in a precise manner. During a muscle activity, many enzymes are released, which control the complex interactions between muscle fibers. Creatine Kinase is the most important enzyme in muscles, which provides essential energy to muscles in the form of ATP.

These ATPs (adenosine triphosphates) are essential energy packets that are utilized when a muscle requires energy for its action. All of our enzymes work in the presence of water, and if our bodies are not hydrated enough, the actions of these enzymes cannot be accomplished. In a dehydrated state, creatine kinase cannot work properly, which leads to a severe energy crisis in our muscles. This, in turn, leads to severely painful muscle knots and muscle tightness. Moreover, a dehydrated muscle is not flexible enough, and it is very prone to injuries.

Thus, a healthy person should drink 3-4 liters of water daily. It is not only essential for muscles but also for our other crucial organs like the brain, heart, liver, stomach, etc. Dehydration leads to inflammation in our body, and toxic materials can slow the recovery of our muscles after a long, hectic day. This is why it is so important to stay hydrated, especially with myofascial pain.

13.Prevention of Myofascial Pains

Throughout this book, I have covered many ways to prevent and treat your myofascial pains. Here is a summary of preventions below. This does not mean that if you do all of the points below, that you will not have myofascial pain, but these methods can go a long way in improving your pains and daily life.

- Eat a balanced diet that incorporates all the macro and micronutrients in calculated amounts.
- Maintain proper posture throughout the day.
- Perform at least 30 minutes of exercise daily.
- Sleep properly to prevent muscle injury.
- Avoid jerky and uncontrolled movements.
- Stay active to maintain proper metabolism in the body.
- Avoid stress and anxieties.
- Focus on positive aspects of life.
- Do yoga and stretching regularly to prevent muscle tightness.
- Do resistance training 3-4 times a week.
- Always know the limits of your muscles.
- Stay hydrated.
- Learn self-treatments for myofascial pain so that you can do an early diagnosis to prevent the worsening of the symptoms.

Important study material for self-learning

Websites

Below are a few websites and books that might be useful for you in treating myofascial trigger points at home.

Important note: the websites mentioned in this book were live at the time of writing but perhaps will not be when you read this book. This is, of course, out of my control.

• www.triggerpoints.net to check where your trigger points are for your pains.

• To learn more about the John F. Barnes' Myofascial Release Approach or find a therapist in your area (if you are in the US), visit www.myomascialrelease.com or www.morerapists.com.

• To learn more about Rolfing, or to find a therapist in your area, visit www.rolf.org or www.rolfinguk.co.uk/ if you are in the UK.

• Learn how to do self–myofascial release with *Myofascial Stretching: A Guide to Self-Treatment* by Jill Stedronsky and Brenda Pardy.

• Visit www.craniocradle.Com for helpful instructional videos on self–myofascial stretching techniques.

• Thera Cane is a cane-shaped tool that allows you to place deep pressure massage on trigger points in the upper back and neck: www.theracane.com. Amazon also have a huge range of There Cane's.

• To learn about micro-current therapy and find a practitioner, visit www.frequencyspecific.com.

www.personalbestpersonaltraining.com

www.myofascialrelease.com

www.painscience.com

www.yogauonline.com

www.mfrcenter.com

www.londonpainclinic.com

www.experiencelife.com

www.themicrocurrentsite.co.uk

www.healthandcare.co.uk/

Recommended books

To learn more about treating your own trigger points, check out:

Anatomy Trains by Thomas W. Myers

Trigger Point Self-Care Manual by Donna Financo

The Concise Book of Trigger Points by Simeon Niel-Asher.

Healing Through Trigger Point Therapy: A Guide to Fibromyalgia, Myofascial Pain and Dysfunction by Devin J. Starlanyl and John Sharkey

The Trigger Point Therapy Workbook: Your Self-Treatment Guide for Pain Relief by Clair Davies and Amber Davies.

Fascia release and balance by Eric Franklin.

Moving Stretch: Work Your Fascia to Free Your Body by Suzanne Wylde.

The Posture Pain Fix: How to Fix Your Back, Neck and Other Postural Problems That Cause Pain in Your Body by Rosalind Ferry.

Life After Pain: 6 Keys to Break Free of Chronic Pain and Get Your Life Back by Dr Jonathan Kuttner.

Mindfulness: A Practical Guide to Finding Peace in a Frantic World by Mark Williams.

Living Pain Free: Healing Chronic Pain with Myofascial Release by Amanda Oswald.

Published by AAV Publishing 2020

Printed in Great Britain
by Amazon

40652024R00066